YIN YOGA THERAPY
AND MENTAL HEALTH

of related interest

Yoga of Recovery
Integrating Yoga and Ayurveda with Modern Recovery Tools for Addiction
Durga Leela
ISBN 978 1 78775 755 4
eISBN 978 1 78775 756 1

Teen Yoga for Yoga Therapists
A Guide to Development, Mental Health and Working with Common Teen Issues
Charlotta Martinus
Foreword by Sir Anthony Seldon
ISBN 978 1 84819 399 4
eISBN 978 0 85701 355 2

Yoga and Science in Pain Care
Treating the Person in Pain
Edited by Neil Pearson, Shelly Prosko and Marlysa Sullivan
Foreword by Timothy McCall
ISBN 978 1 84819 397 0
eISBN 978 0 85701 354 5

YIN YOGA THERAPY AND MENTAL HEALTH

AN INTEGRATED APPROACH

TRACEY MEYERS, PSY.D.

FOREWORD BY SARAH POWERS
ILLUSTRATED BY JENNY SCHNEIDER

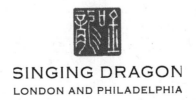

SINGING DRAGON
LONDON AND PHILADELPHIA

First published in Great Britain in 2022 by Singing Dragon, an imprint of Jessica Kingsley Publishers
An imprint of Hodder & Stoughton Ltd
An Hachette Company

1

Copyright © Tracey Meyers, Psy.D. 2022
Foreword copyright © Sarah Powers 2022

A CIP catalogue record for this title is available from the British Library and the Library of Congress

ISBN 978 1 84819 415 1
eISBN 978 0 85701 383 5

Printed and bound in the United States by Integrated Books International

Jessica Kingsley Publishers' policy is to use papers that are natural, renewable, and recyclable products and made from wood grown in sustainable forests. The logging and manufacturing processes are expected to conform to the environmental regulations of the country of origin.

Jessica Kingsley Publishers
Carmelite House
50 Victoria Embankment
London EC4Y 0DZ

www.singingdragon.com

CONTENTS

PART 2: YIN YOGA AND MENTAL HEALTH PRACTICES

FOREWORD

The everlasting nature of Yoga's influence continues to wrap itself in whatever guise it needs to, making its way through time and space into healing various cultures, generations, and populations. Although originated in India many moons ago, methods of holistic body/heart/mind integration continue to pass from teacher to student, forest to city, Sanskrit to English, adept to scientist in ways never imagined millennia ago. From the 5th century BC, when the Buddha's wife may have practiced "yogic temple exercises," to today's gyms, yoga schools, and online apps, people have sought out yoga for a multitude of reasons. Whether we seek to heal an injury, strengthen our immune system, unwind our heavy hearts, or cool our manic minds, yoga has shape shifted again and again, continuing to benefit beings in its constant capacity for reincarnation.

In modernity, most of yoga's marketability can be traced through the fitness community who popularized a low-impact source of physical wellness that promised strength and flexibility to those willing to practice regularly. Although born in caves, monasteries, and ashrams of ancient times, this new form of yoga focused on two main limbs of a multidimensional system: body and breath. Freed of the religious and esoteric depths of its history, yoga grew swiftly in the West, eventually swinging back into vogue and spreading again in the East as well, where secret societies of committed practitioners had never left it.

Although its sports-minded youthful popularity gave it commonality, yoga has always offered itself as an elixir for the mystery minded. Tuning in to the secret messages of one's body/mind intelligence can be found in many esoteric schools of personal transformation. The unique feature of the physical system of yoga that can be learned by almost anyone, children included, is that even when one's motivation for practice is unclear or even superficial, after a short time, a quality of bodily self-awareness and increased personal ease in one's own skin, coupled with a consciousness about healthier living, seems to grow from one's depths. Of course, so much is dependent on how we are taught this inner art of somatic attention, and whether we learn to take care of the parts of us that seek certain results through striving, or that give up easily and become despondent. A proper guide through the world of yoga can empower so many areas of healing within the aspirant, from body-based to mind-blowing. I have seen countless times how yoga can become an ever-growing healing template for how to live artfully with the seas of change within oneself, and our world.

In her therapeutic work as a psychologist, her research as a neuroscientist, as an avid yoga and meditation practitioner and teacher, and now, in writing *Yin Yoga Therapy and Mental Health*, Tracey Meyers has pioneered another dimension of yoga's capacity to touch the lives of those less likely to be exposed to this ancient art of well-being. With her long love of body/mind healing modalities married to her detailed scientific training and layered with her big-heartedness as a psychotherapist, Tracey is the quintessential bridge between these often disparate worlds of influence. With a non-pathologizing approach, Tracey shares stories and accounts, studies, and in-depth research of how yoga and meditation (particularly a meditative style called yin yoga, and mindfulness) have deeply transformed the lives of clients she and others have patiently and lovingly worked with.

I love how Tracey can instruct us in the science behind her experiential insights in such an engaging way; from unpacking such timely themes as the polyvagal theory, eudaimonic well-being, cognitive behavioral therapy, IFS, ANTS, and working with trauma and post-traumatic stress disorder, to the inner methods of breath practices of *pranayama,* postural acuity, visualizations, contemplations, and Buddhist meditations. Without eschewing the essentials of medications, with this integrative approach and psychoeducation, Tracey has expertly opened the floodgates to working in this holistic way with anxiety, depression, nervous system regulation, and even schizophrenia. Through her long hours of study and practice, as a psychological scientist and body/mind teacher, Tracey compassionately welcomes yoga into its natural new home in hospitals and institutions for the modern scientific era. I am sure the shape shifter called yoga certainly won't mind being given yet another impeccable boost of immortality.

Sarah Powers
July 2021

ACKNOWLEDGMENTS

This book reflects my lifelong study of psychology, mindfulness, and yoga along with over 20 years of clinical experience and my own spiritual path. I offer deep gratitude to my many teachers, professors, mentors, clients, and spiritual friends that I continue to learn from on both a personal and professional level.

To my "beshert" (which is Yiddish for soulmate), my husband David, your unending support, encouragement, optimism, and positivity has gotten me through some of the most challenging times not just with this book, but in life. I am so grateful that we get to spend the next half of our lives sharing the beauty and mystery of the world together.

To my beloved children, Jacob, Samantha, and Zoe, I could not be prouder of the three of you and how each of you are on your own path to make the world a better place. Being a mom is the most important job I have, and I love you all so much. To my parents, Gloria and Harry, you have been a steady, loving presence through all of life's ups and downs. Your love for each other and your family has helped me become the person I am now.

To my many friends, teachers, and mentors, I can't begin to thank you for your life lessons, patience, and inspiration. Marlysa Sullivan, my spiritual sister, friend, and colleague, who introduced me to Singing Dragon and believed that I could write this book; Jude Kochman and Pat Harkins, my running partners on the trail and in life; my colleagues at Connecticut Valley Hospital and Department of Mental Health and Addictions, Diane Finlayson and the Maryland University of Integrative Health Yoga Therapy faculty and students; and my teachers, Sarah and Ty Powers, for your support, teachings, wisdom, and love; Richard Miller, Tara Brach, Jack Kornfield, John and Jennifer Welwood, Gregory Kramer, Richard Schwartz, Marsha Linehan, Paul Grilley, and many others.

I would also like to express my sincere appreciation to those who helped me make this book a reality, including Debra Black for your rich writing wisdom; Rachel Feingold for your willingness to jump in and efficiently edit so thoughtfully and professionally; Jenny Schneider who provided the illustrations for this book and made each pose come alive with your compassionate, creative, and openhearted vision of yin yoga; Claire Wilson at Singing Dragon for your patience, kindness, and warm-hearted embrace of yoga and mental health; and a deep bow to my clients that I have had the honor of accompanying on their mental health recovery journeys. I am incredibly grateful to witness the human spirit that you all embody on a daily basis.

INTRODUCTION

It's no secret that there's a growing mental health crisis in our society. Traditional psychiatric treatment has failed to meet the increasing needs of people suffering from myriad mental health conditions; therefore, the search for more innovative and comprehensive treatment has taken on a sense of urgency. Further, turmoil from the past several years, including the global pandemic, political upheavals, and the climate crisis, has contributed to a society coping with higher-than-ever levels of anxiety, trauma, and depression. Consider these statistics from the National Institutes of Health[1] and the Centers for Disease Control and Prevention (CDC):[2]

- Nearly one in five US adults or 51.5 million people (20.6%) in the US experience mental illness in a given year.[3]
- During the global pandemic in 2020–2021, the percentage of adults meeting criteria for anxiety and depression skyrocketed to close to 41.5%.[4]
- The percentage of those reporting an *unmet* mental health need during the global pandemic increased from 9.2% to 11.7%, with young adults and marginalized groups disproportionately affected.[5]

In the last few years, yoga has been more widely studied and accepted as an adjunct mental health treatment. But many therapists aren't exactly sure how to incorporate yoga into their therapeutic tool kit. They don't know which kind of yoga to use, when to use it, or how to use it. The same is true with people suffering from mental health conditions. They often are told to find a yoga class to help them with their mood regulation. They know that yoga is supposed to help them feel better. However, they struggle to figure out what kind of yoga to practice and what would actually help them to feel better.

Yin Yoga Therapy and Mental Health: An Integrative Approach answers those questions. It explores how simple and accessible body-based yoga practices in general—and yin yoga in particular—can be an integral part of a larger holistic approach to reducing emotional pain and improving quality of life for those suffering from mental health issues. *Yin Yoga Therapy and Mental Health* shows readers how to apply the principles of these practices, in combination with different mindfulness and therapeutic techniques, to assist in the treatment of specific mental health conditions, such as stress-related anxiety, depression, and trauma, as well as other severe psychiatric and persistent organic brain disorders, including traumatic brain injury and schizophrenia.

This book is meant to connect yoga and psychotherapy by demonstrating evidence-based approaches to working with clients from both a yoga therapy and a psychotherapy perspective. *Yin Yoga Therapy and Mental Health* will demonstrate how to use yoga poses, meditation, breath work, and psychological methods to decrease emotional suffering and increase self-compassion. Throughout this book, I use real examples of how yin can support well-being for individuals with all types of mental health challenges. To protect their privacy and confidentiality, I utilized composite characters based on the experiences of several of my clients that I have worked with over 25 years. Their experiences are real, as is their yin yoga-based transformational healing. I have created yin sequences and meditation practices that correspond with the theme from each chapter. They can be found in Chapter 16.

ENDNOTES

1   National Institute of Mental Health Statistics on Mental Illness. www.nimh.nih.gov/health/statistics/mental-illness.
2   Vahratian, A., Blumberg, S.J., Terlizzi, E.P., and Schiller, J.S. (2021) 'Symptoms of anxiety or depressive disorder and use of mental health care among adults during the COVID-19 pandemic—United States, August 2020–February 2021.' *MMWR Morbidity and Mortality Weekly Report 2021*, 70, 490–494.
3   National Institute of Mental Health Statistics on Mental Illness. www.nimh.nih.gov/health/statistics/mental-illness.
4   Vahratian, A., Blumberg, S.J., Terlizzi, E.P., and Schiller, J.S. (2021) 'Symptoms of anxiety or depressive disorder and use of mental health care among adults during the COVID-19 pandemic—United States, August 2020–February 2021.' *MMWR Morbidity and Mortality Weekly Report 2021*, 70, 490–494.
5   Vahratian, A., Blumberg, S.J., Terlizzi, E.P., and Schiller, J.S. (2021) 'Symptoms of anxiety or depressive disorder and use of mental health care among adults during the COVID-19 pandemic—United States, August 2020–February 2021.' *MMWR Morbidity and Mortality Weekly Report 2021*, 70, 490–494.

— Part 1 —

YIN YOGA AND MENTAL HEALTH FOUNDATIONS

— Chapter 1 —

WHAT IS YIN YOGA?

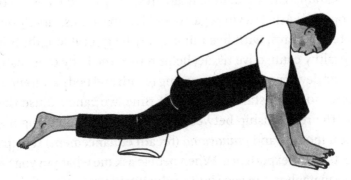

*Dragon can be a challenging pose for many yin students, yet it
can support their ability to stay with discomfort*

The first time I ever took a yin yoga class, I didn't like it at all. The teacher led
us into Dragon, a deep knee-down lunge, and invited us to fold forward over
one knee and rest on our fingertips for the next five minutes. After only a few
breaths, I began to feel agitated. How could I possibly stay still for the next
five minutes, never mind an entire class? Sweat poured off me onto my yoga
mat. I wanted to pack it up and bolt. But just so I wouldn't embarrass myself,
I resolved to stay in the pose, get through the class, and never do this again. I
tried my best to breathe, relax, and soften as the teacher suggested. I took furtive
glances around the room to see if other people were hating this as much as I
was. But everyone looked calm and relaxed. Could they actually be enjoying
this? Impossible! Soften and relax? No way. After five minutes, which felt like
an hour, a meditation bell chimed, and the teacher guided us out of the pose
and into Child's pose. I immediately felt calmer. Being in this pose was a very
different experience. It was like a do-over in Little League. Maybe this wouldn't
be so bad after all!

Pose after pose, I watched as my inner experiences shifted—my emotions,
energy, thoughts, and physical body—depending on the shape we were in and

my response to what I was observing. By the time class was over, I felt alive and energized, open to my emotions just as I experienced them. I was hooked.

In the past ten years, I have plunged deeper and deeper into yin yoga. I went on to do advanced trainings, studying with master yin yoga teachers including Paul Grilley and Sarah and Ty Powers. I earned my 500-hour certification in Insight Yoga with Sarah Powers, one of the founding teachers of yin yoga; I became a certified yoga therapist. I developed my own yin yoga training for yoga teachers and saw how it benefited them, both in their teaching and in their own lives.

Yin, a relatively new form of yoga compared to older styles such as Ashtanga, Iyengar, or Bikram, is now taught in mainstream yoga studios across the United States, Europe, and Asia.[1] In yin yoga, we hold simple poses, largely on the floor, for one to ten minutes, with five minutes as the typical length; this practice promotes healthy connective tissue, helps return the body to its natural range of motion, and develops mindfulness using breath and body awareness. Because we hold poses for a substantial period of time, we can also use the practice to cultivate the relationship between the mind and body using meditation, psychological inquiry, and *pranayama* (breath enhancement) to explore more subtle aspects of the experience. When people ask me what yin yoga is, I like to give a simple metaphor. Yin yoga is like tofu: it takes the shape, form, color, and taste of the ingredients that are applied to it. It can be a deep physical practice, a form of mindfulness meditation, or a compassionate way to work through emotional pain.

HOW DOES YIN DIFFER FROM OTHER FORMS OF YOGA?

There are several important distinctions between yin yoga and other forms of traditional yoga (the most common found in the US include Hatha, Vinyasa, Ashtanga, Iyengar, and Bikram). First, yin poses are held for longer, and often an entire class will include only five to ten poses, while a Hatha yoga practice might include upwards of 25 poses.

Second, yin yoga differs from other forms of yoga in terms of its basic instructions. In a Hatha yoga class, an instructor might suggest to "engage, elongate, reach, stretch, activate" when describing how to enter into a pose or maintain a pose for a prescribed period, usually under a minute. In a yin yoga class, instructions are rooted in the idea that one must "soften," "relax into," "load," or "stress." Yin instructions are less alignment-based. In other words, in yin we are not worried about whether toes are turned out or under, whether the hips are up in the air or sitting on the heels. Instead, the instructions are provided only as guidance; the student is the one to determine what feels best for their particular body. For example, if a yin teacher is leading a child pose in a yin class, they may emphasize softening and letting go into the pose, providing props like blankets or a bolster if there are fragile areas of the body like knees or hips, and encouraging the student to take a shape that works for their body.

Third, sometimes yin yoga is confused with other, quieter practices like restorative yoga because of the occasional use of props. However, in restorative yoga, the connective tissue is not being stressed or "loaded," but rather the props are used to open the body in a very gentle way. In yin, we might use propping if there is an area of the body that is fragile, injured, or prohibiting us from getting into the pose we would like due to compression which causes a bone-on-bone restriction preventing more mobility, but we are still loading the connective tissues through pressurizing them over time. Props help to keep us in the pose by easing discomfort and protecting from injury, while still allowing active loading of the connective tissue.

Fourth, we are not trying to move our bodies into poses or shapes that match an ideal yoga prototype. Canadian yoga teacher Bernie Clark (2012) shares this lovely quote that I find to be very helpful around this idea. He says, "We don't use our body to get into a pose, we use the pose to get into our body."[2] This shift from trying to imitate the yoga teacher or trying to look like the other students in the room to developing personalized practice is what I like to refer to as "non-competitive yoga." Students can learn to drop the judging, evaluating, and often self-critical stories that keep them from enjoying yoga (and many other things in life for that matter) and become interested in how the shapes affect their body in that particular moment in time. As a yoga student myself, I found this to be liberating. In the 15 years that I have been practicing yoga, there have been so many times that I would leave a yoga class feeling disappointed in myself that I could not "achieve" a certain pose. I would sometimes transfer that disappointment into anger toward myself. These thoughts would take over and replay again and again: "I am not a good yoga student," "How can I teach yoga if I can't even do this pose?" and even "I hate my body." For people who struggle with mental health issues, negative thoughts can often lead to an increase in depression, anxiety, or despair. So, if these feelings are coming up in a yoga practice, it can create dis-ease rather than comfort and support. Yin yoga provides relief from these negative and critical judgments because we are not trying to measure up to an ideal body type. Yin allows us to investigate rather than evaluate; open rather than close down; find freedom instead of fixation on the negative.

Yin yoga, as we practice it today, began in the late 1990s and early 2000s through a collaboration between yoga teacher pioneers Paul Grilley and Sarah Powers, along with Dr. Motoyama, a yoga master/healer from Japan.[3] I have had the good fortune to study with both Paul and Sarah, who have inspired thousands of students and teachers to incorporate yin yoga into their regular practice. Paul is a scholar of yoga, anatomy, and meridian theory, which he combined to create yin yoga. He emphasizes how yin yoga can "gently stretch and rehabilitate the connective tissues that form our joints."[4] He also emphasizes muscular and skeletal variations that are unique to each person. He has an illuminating website with pictures of actual cadaver bones that show variations.[5] Paul has shifted conventional thinking about teaching yoga from emphasizing how all students should look the same in a pose to an individualized practice that is safe and appropriate for one's own unique structure.

Sarah Powers learned yin as a student of Paul's in the early 1980s. With her strong background in psychology and Buddhist meditation studies, she found that the practice offered her a natural platform to explore mindfulness and other psychological methods. She studied with Dr. Motoyama and learned about Traditional Chinese Medicine and meridian theory. From her studies, she investigated how certain poses can stimulate "meridians" throughout the body, opening blockages in the physical, emotional, and energetic realms, and creating balance between body and mind.

Powers writes, "The Meridian Theory posited by many masters, such as Dr. Hiroshi Motoyama and his student Paul Grilley, suggests that the connective tissues of the body house a liquid-rich and highly sensitive energy system that can be influenced positively by the way the body is treated."[6] She coined the term *yin* yoga, weaving together the practices and philosophies of Yoga, Buddhism, and psychological investigation. Sarah is a master yoga and meditation teacher and has a huge following around the world. She and her husband Ty, a meditation teacher and deep spiritual practitioner, created the Insight Yoga Institute, an advanced teacher training program that has been instrumental in my own development as a yoga practitioner and teacher and as a therapist.[7]

BASIC PRINCIPLES OF YIN YOGA

Guiding principles for yin yoga therapy must emphasize safety and stability to establish the foundation for transformational healing.

PRINCIPLE 1: TAKE THE SHAPE AND FIND AN APPROPRIATE LEVEL OF DEPTH AND SENSATION

When the body comes into a new shape, the first reaction will be to engage the muscle fibers to automatically protect the ligaments and joints. This is what I call the "first edge." Once the body recognizes that it is safe to stay in the shape, which usually takes 60 to 90 seconds to fully adjust to the sensations, the muscle fibers ease off and there is more direct access to the deeper connective tissues. That is why holding a pose for at least one minute is key. Shorter than that, the body will remain more muscularly engaged and the connective tissues will not get stimulated directly. After the 60 to 90 seconds, we begin to experience the sensations of the tissues being stimulated, and often it is possible to move deeper into the pose.

We may not always choose to move deeper into the pose. Sometimes, just mild sensation is appropriate, especially for new students. Strong sensations can cause all sorts of physical and emotional reactions in the mind and/or body. Like my Dragon experience in my first class, students can be caught off guard by the intensity of the sensations, especially if they are in a pose for an extended period. When this happens, they may come off the pose early, or they may "grit their teeth" and get through it, but never want to come back to my class!

When I teach, I begin gradually, allowing students to find their own "edge" for each particular pose in each particular moment. I often ask students to use a Likert scale I developed from one to ten, anchored with the following metrics: 1 = no sensation/neutral; 5 = deep sensation (sometimes like a dull ache or a pulling sensation); 10 = pain (sharp, shooting, or nerve).

I advise students to immediately come out of the pose if they are any higher than a seven, as something may be injured or unstable. As students begin a practice, I ask them to find a place on this scale, somewhere between a two and a five, that they can stay with for a period of time. This intensity might change within the pose as a few minutes pass, or it might be a completely different experience the next time they do the pose. Rather than trying to strive toward a higher "edge" number, I invite students to find a sensation that is *interesting* and allows them to investigate without getting restless or significantly uncomfortable. I find that giving them a scale or incremental approach is helpful in figuring out what is best for their body. Ultimately, this provides an internal sense of safety as the student can regulate the depth and intensity of the pose.

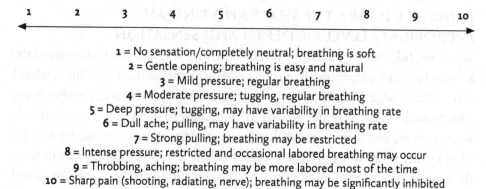

1 = No sensation/completely neutral; breathing is soft
2 = Gentle opening; breathing is easy and natural
3 = Mild pressure; regular breathing
4 = Moderate pressure; tugging, regular breathing
5 = Deep pressure; tugging, may have variability in breathing rate
6 = Dull ache; pulling, may have variability in breathing rate
7 = Strong pulling; breathing may be restricted
8 = Intense pressure; restricted and occasional labored breathing may occur
9 = Throbbing, aching; breathing may be more labored most of the time
10 = Sharp pain (shooting, radiating, nerve); breathing may be significantly inhibited

Yin sensation scale

SENSATION INQUIRY

Notice where the sensation is.

Notice the intensity of the sensation (use of scale above).

Notice qualities of the sensation (does it have shape, color, movement?).

Notice if the sensation changes over the duration of the pose.

Notice if there are accompanying feelings or emotions along with the sensation.

PRINCIPLE 2: TARGET THE CONNECTIVE TISSUE RATHER THAN THE MUSCLES

Usually after a breath or two, students will begin to feel some discomfort—and then name what they feel in their bodies. Often it feels like tight or stiff muscles, soreness, and so on. What's really happening is fascial thickness, tension, or compression. In contrast to a more conventional, active yoga practice that emphasizes movement through rhythmic stretching of the muscles, yin yoga targets the connective tissues of the body by loading and compressing in static positions. Of course, there is going to be some muscular engagement in many yin poses as well, due to the connections between connective tissue and muscles, but the emphasis is much more directly on the connective tissue.

Connective tissues are found throughout the body and include bone, blood, cartilage, tendons, ligaments, and fascia—which is deeply embedded within the tissues and connects the body below the surface of the skin. Fascia has drawn significant interest over the past decade, with a growing body of evidence showing how important it is for our overall flexibility and movement.[8,9] There are many comprehensive resources that give in-depth descriptions of fascia and connective tissue that are beyond the scope of this book. I would highly recommend Tom Myers's book *Anatomy Trains*[10] and David Lesondak's book *Fascia: What It Is and Why It Matters.*[11]

By gently stimulating or stressing the connective tissues, we can provide joint support along with bone strengthening. Studies in physical therapy and other rehabilitation methods that use positions akin to yin poses have shown that low-force stretching can produce long-lasting results in terms of range of motion, pain reduction, and a better healing response.[12] To understand how low-force stretching can produce results, Paul Grilley and others have utilized the metaphor of braces. Those of us who suffered through adolescence with braces will recall the seemingly endless months required for the braces to move the teeth into proper alignment. However, over time, the gentle and persistent pressure changes and realigns the teeth. This is the same underlying principle of yin yoga. Connective tissue does not respond to stretching and movement as our muscles do. That is why even when we exercise regularly through Hatha yoga or aerobic activity, we may feel stiff and inflexible as we age because we are not impacting the connective tissue and supporting the health of the joints. Yin yoga, on the other hand, specifically targets the connective tissue, allowing for increased moisture, particularly of synovial fluid in the joint capsules and rehydration of the fascial matrix. In his book *Yinsights,* Bernie Clark discusses in depth the benefit of stressing the connective tissue "in an intelligent and safe way, to targeted areas of the body."[13] He describes how yin yoga can keep the collagen fibers and the ground substances (gel-like fluids) functioning properly to lubricate, protect, and support the tissues and joints of the body, so that toxins and waste are eliminated and our bodies move with more ease and fluidity even as we age.

To know how long to hold a pose—and even what an "edge" means—students need to know the difference between tension and compression, and between pain and discomfort. To target the connective tissue and find an appropriate depth to move into, it is important for beginning yin students to notice the difference between tension and compression. In a yin pose, we are intentionally cultivating "tension," or the sensation of pulling and tugging on the connective tissue. Over time, the body learns to slowly release tension, allowing for increased flexibility and mobility of the joints. This can happen even within a five-minute pose, but usually requires an ongoing practice.

However, there are times where the body will simply not be able to move further into a pose no matter how long one holds it. This indicates that compression is occurring. Compression refers to the restriction in the body's skeletal system such that when a person moves into a particular pose, bones are meeting other bones or are pressuring the tissue directly and there is no room for further movement. As Paul Grilley brilliantly points out in his pictures of bones, we all have different skeletal systems made up of different sized and shaped bones that impact each of us differently. When two bones meet each other, there is no range of motion available. Forcing further movement can cause injury. That is another reason why we move slowly into a pose and determine whether there is more range of motion or if we have met compression. Compression can feel painful or can be experienced simply as the absence of space to move further into the pose. Then, it is time to adjust and find a different variation of the pose or use props—or simply dial back from the pose and enjoy the sensations prior to reaching compression. We can learn to stay with varying degrees of sensation in our yin yoga practice (our "edge" for the pose) depending on our body's structure, how we are feeling emotionally, and where we want to stimulate particular areas of the body.

PRINCIPLE 3: DIVE INTO STILLNESS

Stillness is often the biggest challenge for new students, who are used to moving from pose to pose with little time to pause and reflect on what is happening. Yin asks them to come into a pose and then just stay still and do nothing. Students can get restless and uncomfortable staying still after a relatively short time. They may start shifting in their bodies, looking around the room, unsure of what they should be doing. I even had a student once who had his phone next to him and would sneak glances at it during yin poses. That is where the teacher plays a significant role in guiding students during these still periods, because staying in relative stillness (with the ability to make small physical adjustments as needed while in the shape, including the depth of the pose, the rate of the breath, or adding in a prop for support) is therapeutic not only for the body, as we learned above, but also for the mind.

During stillness, a teacher can guide students to attend to different aspects of the mind and body. This may include specific instructions on working with the mind, teachings around topics related to physical sensations, or developing more compassion toward oneself. This integration of wisdom teachings can make yin yoga a deep dive into an integrative path of healing. You don't have to be an expert in any of these traditions to be able to integrate some of the teachings into a particular pose or series of poses. For example, each of these traditions utilizes meditation as part of its practice that can be incorporated while the student is in the pose. For beginning students, I will spend time focusing on the basics of mindfulness meditation. This helps students to have something to focus their minds on, relaxing some of the repetitive and often negative self-talk and keeping them interested and engaged in the practice. There are excellent books that break down mindfulness into simple and easy-to-understand directions that can be utilized within a yin class. I like to use the following sources for mindfulness: *Mindfulness in Plain English,*[14] *Full Catastrophe Living,*[15] and *Breath by Breath,*[16] to teach students the basics of mindfulness in each pose.

This first chapter has focused on demystifying yin yoga and identifying what it really is and what it is not. Yin yoga is a deeper, more integrative platform than traditional forms of yoga that can be utilized to help people who are suffering or just want to feel more alive and happier. It is body-based, but integrates mindfulness, meditation, and psychological methods. Meditation and psychological work can be very hard for people, particularly those with mental health issues. Yin yoga gets people out of their thinking minds and into their bodies, which can help them learn self-regulation and allow them to develop the tools for healing. I believe that yin is the next generation of yoga for mental health. Over the next chapters, you will learn how to use yin yoga to help those who are on a healing journey.

ENDNOTES

1   Leviton, R. (1990) 'Yoga in America.' *Yoga Journal, 91,* 40–101. www.beezone.com/Yogain-America/yoga_in_america.html. CreateSpace Independent Publishing Platform.
2   Clark, B. (2012) *The Complete Guide to Yin Yoga.* Ashland, OR: White Cloud Press.
3   Grilley, P. (2012) *Yin Yoga Principles and Practice* (10th anniversary ed.). Ashland, OR: White Cloud Press.
4   Grilley, P., and Grilley, S. (2021) Yoga Studies. Bone Photos. www.paulgrilley.com/bones.
5   Grilley, P., and Grilley, S. (2021) Yoga Studies. Bone Photos. www.paulgrilley.com/bones.
6   Powers, S. (2008) *Insight Yoga.* Boulder, CO: Shambhala Publications, p.13.
7   www.sarahpowers.com
8   Schleip, R. (2017) *Fascial Fitness: How to be resilient, elegant and dynamic in everyday life and sport.* Chichester, UK: Lotus Publishing.
9   Page, P. (2012) 'Current concepts in muscle stretching for exercise and rehabilitation.' *International Journal of Sports Physical Therapy, 7,* 1, 109–119. www.ncbi.nlm.nih.gov/pmc/articles/PMC3273886.
10 Myers, T. (2014) *Anatomy Trains* (3rd ed.). London: Churchill Livingston.
11 Lesondak, D. (2017) *Fascia: What it is and why it matters.* London: Handspring Publishers.
12 Page, P. (2012) 'Current concepts in muscle stretching for exercise and rehabilitation.' *International Journal of Sports Physical Therapy, 7,* 1, 109–119. www.ncbi.nlm.nih.gov/pmc/articles/PMC3273886.
13 Clark, B. (2007) *Yinsights.* Creative Independent Publishing Platform.
14 Gunaratana, B. (2011) *Mindfulness in Plain English.* Bloomington, IN: Wisdom Publishers.
15 Zinn-Kabat, J. (2013) *Full Catastrophe Living.* New York: Bantam Publishers.
16 Rosenberg, L. (2004) *Breath by Breath.* Boston, MA: Shambhala Publishers.

— Chapter 2 —

YIN YOGA

An Integrative Healing Approach

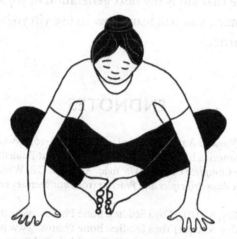

Butterfly pose can create a sense of openness in the physical and emotional body by staying connected to the subtle, yet persistent sensations

An increasing number of mental health therapists are seeking mind-body approaches to treat mental health problems, having come up against what they see are the limitations of conventional psychiatry. Their clients demand it; they want (and need) better options than what they've been given. My own clients admit they're tired of the groups, medications, and same-old, same-old treatments they've been offered—sometimes for years. The good news is that yoga and mindful awareness practices have increasingly found their way into therapy offices, hospital settings, and group homes—and researchers are more eager than in the past to study the effects. Unfortunately, so far, such approaches have been consigned to the status of adjunct therapies—what the medical establishment calls "complementary and alternative medicine"—rather than specific healing or therapeutic methods, at least until they "prove" themselves. Hopefully, as the body of research increases, the role of yoga therapy will expand and become an integral part of a new holistic medicine paradigm instead of merely an adjunct or even an elective practice.

While yoga may be a relative newcomer in Western mental health therapy, it established its credentials and proved itself at least 2000 years ago. The *Yoga Sutras* of Patanjali, probably compiled around the 2nd century CE, is one of the most important, and certainly the most well known, of the ancient yoga texts. The Sutras provide powerful tools to help alleviate suffering, including meditation, breathing practices, and physical postures. Over 2000 years later, people continue to turn toward yoga when they experience physical pain, emotional distress, or spiritual disconnection.[1] I hear this in my public yoga classes, where students most often admit that they come to class because they're stressed out, anxious, depressed, or they want to relax. My clients who are hospitalized are also interested in yoga. They have heard that yoga and meditation can help them feel better. And they want that, especially those who feel that their previous treatment did not help enough.

I must admit I didn't know much about yoga when I started working as a conventional clinical psychologist in psychiatric and rehabilitation centers. My area of interest was neuropsychology, the relationship between the brain and behavior using assessment measures, clinical observation, and cognitive-behavioral techniques—a far cry from a mind-body-spirit approach! Many of my clients had significant cognitive impairment brought on by mental illness, such as schizophrenia and traumatic brain injury; side-effects from medications; traumatic events, including repeated adverse events in early childhood including trauma, exposure to violence, and broken homes; and developmental disorders such as autism. These problems included difficulty with concentration, new learning, memory, judgment, impulse control, and problem-solving. So, it stands to reason that cognitive behavioral "talk therapy"—with its emphasis on new learning, verbal reasoning, and memory—wasn't very successful in fostering sustainable behavioral changes. Many of my clients weren't able to understand, recall, or integrate into everyday life the skills I was teaching. While they appreciated the opportunity to talk about their issues to a compassionate listener, they didn't seem to feel any more empowered or capable of healing their emotional pain after working with me than before. I began to doubt my own abilities as a psychologist and to lose faith in our whole approach to psychiatric treatment in the West.

And then I met Jim.

Jim had sustained a severe traumatic brain injury when he was 32 and was on a long recovery journey by the time I met him five years later. He had progressed from a wheelchair to a walker, from a walker to a cane, and, finally, to walking unassisted. He had learned to talk again through speech therapy and, although his speech was often hard to understand, he was able to communicate verbally. He had reached the point of needing only limited verbal prompts for dressing, bathing, and eating. However, he still had profound memory impairment, impulse control issues, and poor emotional regulation. His physiatrist referred Jim to me to work on anger management, social skills training, and ultimately to help him develop positive and meaningful relationships.

Alas, after two years of working together, it was clear that Jim had reached a plateau in his overall recovery. His behavior, while improved, was still impulsive. His balance was off, and he walked with a shuffling gait. He still struggled with emotional outbursts, often yelling at his caregivers and expressing deep sorrow about "losing my life." His clinical team brainstormed, and we came up with a plan of action that included a few "out of the box" suggestions. One of them was to recommend a local yoga therapist who could address his balance and his mind-body awareness, and offer him some calming strategies. He began an intensive one-on-one program with the yoga therapist, meeting her once a week and augmenting that with a home practice three times a week. Over the following six months, he made great progress. His walking and his posture improved; he no longer looked down when he was outdoors, and the slump in his shoulders disappeared. His yoga sessions impacted our time together as well. He was calmer and more focused, able to converse and maintain eye contact with me for the first time. Yoga helped him move beyond what we thought was possible. He continues to practice yoga regularly and has made small but appreciative gains over the last two years.

Jim's experience with yoga got me thinking seriously about whether such a practice would benefit my other clients. But not everyone has access to private yoga therapy sessions, like Jim did. Could yoga be incorporated into individual or group therapy sessions—and if so, to what extent? What if I, as a clinical psychologist, could use yoga to help my clients improve their physical, emotional, and cognitive limitations? That's what I wanted: to be able to offer yoga to my clients to support them in making positive changes in their lives; I was confident that I could do it because yoga had already been instrumental in my own spiritual and healing journey. I had been practicing yoga seriously for five years at that point, and I loved how I felt after taking classes. So, I screwed up my courage and enrolled in a yoga teacher training program, the first step toward becoming a yoga therapist. After nine months of philosophy, poses (*asana*), breathing (*pranayama*), and sequencing, I was ready to take my show on the road and start teaching.

Teaching at a yoga studio was great fun. I learned how to offer different postural cues, direct people to pay attention to their breathing, and provide helpful suggestions for working with the mind. My students learned quickly and enjoyed the challenges as much as I had when I was a student. I felt confident. I was ready to move beyond the studio and offer yoga at the hospital where I worked. I quickly discovered, however, that teaching yoga in a mental health setting was a whole other kettle of fish.

The first community class I taught at the hospital was for clients on a long-term care inpatient psychiatric ward. It didn't quite go as planned. Sure, as a teacher trainee I had learned how to help students orchestrate a pose properly by giving them verbal and physical cues, modifications, and an array of different props to support their bodies. But no one clued me in that teaching psychiatric clients would require infinitely more patience, flexibility, and humor than I could ever imagine.

Luckily, the first class was small. Only four students—inpatient clients all with different cognitive and emotional challenges. I gave them each a brand-new mat, a block, and a strap. Juan, with his devilish grin and a long history of manic behaviors, immediately grabbed the strap and put it around his neck, pretending to strangle himself. Alarmed, I jumped up and grabbed it out of his hand, and quickly retrieved the straps from the other three clients. He assured me that he was only kidding, but I was already doubting the wisdom of my decision.

Another student, a woman who was blind in one eye and very unsteady on her feet, needed my help getting down onto the floor and then up again, interrupting the flow of the class, the sequence I was trying to teach, and my train of thought. After a bit, she asked to be excused to use the bathroom; she never came back. Twenty minutes into class, a bell rang indicating that it was lunch time. Class over. I vowed never to teach again. Later that day, Juan saw me on the unit and asked when we could practice again. "I like that yoga," he told me. "I feel good, you know. More relaxed." Who knew? I kept teaching.

Looking back, I shouldn't have been surprised that yoga helped Juan and others feel "good, you know. More relaxed." But yoga hasn't been traditionally practiced in psychiatric settings, particularly not in inpatient units where doctors subscribe to a reductionist model: stabilize the symptoms through use of psychopharmacology; continue active treatment with more medication, psychotherapy, social skills, and anger management classes—all valuable approaches to be sure. But it doesn't have to stop there. Yoga offers additional benefits, and its usefulness is being studied with greater frequency in the last two decades. Elizabeth Visceglia, MD, a psychiatrist and researcher in New York City, says yoga can improve outcomes in psychiatric clients by "activating a cascade of physiologic and emotional changes and by utilizing the healing power of breath, movement, and awareness of mind and body."[2] Basically, many of these research studies are reporting that yoga plays an important role in balancing the nervous system. According to Patricia Gerbarg, MD, co-author of a study looking at yoga as an adjunct treatment for generalized anxiety disorder, "Restoring sympathovagal balance and resiliency is fundamental to treatment of most disorders seen in psychiatric, pediatric, and general medical practice."[3] In the age of modern medicine and science, research is beginning to show what the ancient and modern yoga students have already known: yoga can be an effective therapy to treat mind-body-spirit.[4, 5, 6]

Yoga therapy as a holistic medical approach has been elucidated beautifully by Dr. Timothy McCall in his seminal textbook, *Yoga as Medicine: The Yogic Prescription for Health and Healing*.[7] He describes how yoga is a "holistic approach" to treating medical problems (including stress-related emotional disorders) rather than the reductionist approach that is most often found in conventional medicine which, according to McCall, "tries to reduce the complexity of illness to one factor, and then tries to attack it with a 'magic bullet'—drugs or surgery."[8] In contrast, yoga therapy is a holistic approach since "holism involves looking at all sides of a problem, and trying to intervene at as many points as possible and as gently as possible."[9] (See Table 2.1 for key differences between yoga and traditional medicine approaches to healing.)

Table 2.1 Different approaches to healing from medical and yoga perspectives

Conventional medicine approach	Yoga as medicine approach
Reductionistic	Holistic
Faster in onset	Slower in onset
Effects tend to wane over time	Effects tend to increase over time
Best at dealing with acute problems (accidents, emergencies)	Less good at dealing with acute problems
Less good at dealing with chronic problems (diabetes, arthritis)	Very good at dealing with chronic problems
Less good at dealing with psychosomatic illness (stress, irritable bowel syndrome, headaches, etc.)	Excellent at dealing with psychosomatic illness
Good at dealing with pain (at least in theory) but poor with suffering	Can help with pain and excellent at dealing with suffering

Therapies usually rely on one major mechanism of action	Therapies rely on many simultaneous mechanisms of action
Treatments are standardized	Treatments are tailored to the individual
Often ignores possible healing synergies	Relies on additive and multiplying effects for synergistic interventions
Side-effects usually negative	Side-effects often positive
Doctor-controlled	Client-controlled
Client is mostly the passive recipient of therapy. Client can be unconscious	Client actively does the treatment (with some guidance). Consciousness required
Usually little learning involved	Involves learning
High tech	Low tech
Many treatments must be given in hospital or clinic	Treatments can be done at home
Disdains anecdotal evidence	Relies on direct experience of client
Relies on diagnostic tests over direct exam of the client	Relies on direct observation of the client
Expensive and may require continued expenditure over time	Inexpensive: once you learn yoga and buy props, is free unless you decide to study more
Minor emphasis on prevention	Major emphasis on prevention
Absence of symptoms or signs of disease and normal lab tests are equated with health	Health is defined as a high level of physical, emotional, and spiritual well-being

(Adapted from *Yoga as Medicine*)[10]

After teaching for quite a while, I had an experience that made me question the type of yoga I was offering inpatient clients. I was teaching a class to a group of clients who were newly admitted to a 45-day substance-abuse treatment program at the hospital where I worked. Most of the clients had never taken yoga before and were, understandably, a bit nervous. One woman, Jesse, looked particularly tired and wary—and very uncomfortable. She positioned herself at the back of the room and announced that she didn't expect to stay for the whole class. She figured she could probably get down onto the floor but wasn't convinced she could get up again. I encouraged her to do only what she felt she could do, or even wanted to do. I would be nearby if she needed me. With her in mind, I chose a floor-based practice, and I began with some meditation, breath work, and a few basic warm-ups, followed by several yin poses. No one had to worry about getting up and down multiple times.

As class went on, I watched Jesse's face brighten. She smiled and nodded as I wove in themes around connecting with the body with kindness. She laughed as she wobbled through a few balancing poses and became noticeably still for the final yin sequence. At the end of class, she gave me a huge hug and announced that this was the best she had felt in years. Her beautiful eyes were soft, bright, and alive. After just *one* practice! Her experience touched me deeply; it was a true testament to how powerful yin yoga can be, especially for those who need self-care so desperately. And yet, I began to think, something was missing for me in teaching traditional Hatha yoga.

WHY YIN?

That day after I taught yin to the clients on the substance-abuse unit, I realized that the yoga I had been teaching limited me to more able-bodied and perhaps more confident students. Yes, it calmed their nervous systems, cleared their minds, and even gave them a better sense of their physical body in space. I had many wonderful experiences with clients like Jim, Jesse, and Juan. But what if I could teach any student who wanted to experience the benefits of yoga and meditation, no matter what their physical or cognitive limitations were? What if I could teach in a way that deeply resonated with the way I see mental health recovery as a whole—as a lifelong journey of opening, softening, and expanding one's capacity to tolerate both discomfort and ease? The answer, of course, was right in front of me: to teach yin yoga in therapeutic settings and train other yoga therapists and clinicians in the foundations of yin so that this powerful and healing modality can expand into diverse therapeutic settings.

Yin yoga is first and foremost a physical practice. If a person cannot do certain poses or activities due to physical limitations, the possibility of benefiting from the practice is quite limited. I am not the kind of teacher who says, if you can't do the pose, just sit out and breathe and watch the class and you will get benefit. To benefit from a yoga practice, students must be able to get into their bodies, to begin to connect with the full range of direct physical sensations and eventually more subtle energies. Yin allows people to get into their bodies without having to worry about balance or flexibility or strength. The poses are accessible with variations and props to physically accommodate most bodies. Even those students who feel extremely self-conscious about stepping on a yoga mat discover that they can feel at home in yin yoga with its emphasis on self-discovery. They don't have to stand up, move around the room, or make eye contact with others, or even with the teacher. Their mat becomes their home base.

Yin is a form of *insight meditation,* allowing people to come into the present moment, see what is going on in their inner world, and create a safe space without harsh self-judgment. For many students, sitting meditation can be extremely difficult, if not next to impossible, especially when they have physical limitations or suffer from mental health issues like anxiety and have racing or discursive thoughts. Yin yoga can be a platform to learn and practice meditation much more easily since they can assume whatever shape works for their body structure, the meditation is brief (up to five minutes) before a new pose is introduced, and they can choose when to come out of the pose and when to shift the focus of their attention. The shift from the teacher setting the parameters for how to do the pose, how to breathe, how to direct the mind to the student creating their own practice makes yin a safe, empowering, and therapeutic form of yoga.

Yin is a subtle body practice, allowing people to feel for themselves the effects of tracking and modulating the breath, the flow of energy in the body, and how the poses might make them feel more awake, alert, and alive—or calm, relaxed, and at ease. Yin becomes an investigation for what happens when they are uncomfortable due to physical sensations. Does the student start to dissociate, get upset, become resistant, or go deeper into the discomfort? No matter which way a person works with discomfort, this becomes a doorway for handling greater challenges off the mat. One of my early meditation teachers, Cheri Huber, has a wonderful Zen quote that I think about often: "How you do anything is how you do everything."[11] Yin teaches students how to discover patterns and work with them through the physical body and meditation, and eventually, how to utilize them as a transformational path in their daily lives.

While yin is physically accessible, easy to teach and learn, and can provide a platform for weaving in psychological and mindfulness work, it is still largely unknown, avoided, or misunderstood by the yoga community, especially regarding its potential benefit for mental health conditions. I recently taught an advanced course in mental health and yoga to yoga teachers in which the majority of the class had never taken more than a few yin classes, did not know how to teach yin, and avoided the practice altogether. When I asked them what their concerns were about teaching yin to their students and clients, the feedback I received was surprising. They said that yin was boring; that it could be very physically uncomfortable; that the silent periods made them feel like they had nothing to offer their students; that they were worried the students might overstretch or destabilize areas of the body; that they had personally tried yin and did not like it or had been injured in some way from yin; that they did not know how to offer modifications; and that they preferred other forms of yoga with which they were much more familiar, including yoga *nidra* (a guided yoga meditation) and restorative yoga.

To challenge some of these beliefs, I led a simple yin sequence and emphasized mindfulness of the breath and provided them with simple instructions: to just notice what was happening at that time. Just as with my clients at the hospital, I provided them with simple guidelines to stay in the pose only as long as it felt safe, to modify and move as appropriate, and to treat each pose as an opportunity to be with themselves in a kind and nurturing way. Following just one class, many of the students—including ones who had had prior negative experiences—shifted their perspective around yin yoga. They liked the fact that they could move, modify poses, and did not have to remain in discomfort. They learned ways to keep their bodies safe if they were either hypermobile or had an injury. They enjoyed hearing the inquiry questions and gentle guidance around meditation, and they were curious about how to integrate yin into their yoga therapy sessions. Soon after the course, several of those students contacted me to let me know that they had integrated yin into their tool kits. Just as my clients had experienced significant benefits from a single yin class, these seasoned yoga teachers had also been transformed after just one yin practice. Quite simply, yin works!

ENDNOTES

1 Büssing, A., Michalsen, A., Khalsa, S.B.S., Telles, S., and Sherman, K.J. (2012) 'Effects of yoga on mental and physical health: A short summary of reviews.' *Evidence-Based Complementary & Alternative Medicine (eCAM).* doi: 10.1155/2012/165410.

2 Visceglia, E., and Lewis, S. (2011) 'Yoga therapy as an adjunctive treatment for schizophrenia: A randomized, controlled pilot study.' *Journal of Alternative and Complementary Medicine, 17,* 7, 601–607.

3 Gerbarg, P. (2017) 'Breathing Techniques in Psychiatric Treatment.' In Gerbarg, P., Muskin, P., and Brown, R. (eds) *Complementary and Integrative Treatments in Psychiatric Practice.* Washington, DC: American Psychiatric Association Publishing, p.241.

4 Büssing, A., Michalsen, A., Khalsa, S.B.S., Telles, S., and Sherman, K.J. (2012) 'Effects of yoga on mental and physical health: A short summary of reviews.' *Evidence-Based Complementary & Alternative Medicine (eCAM).* doi: 10.1155/2012/165410.

5 Cabral, P., Meyer, H.B., and Ames, D. (2011) 'Effectiveness of yoga therapy as a complementary treatment for major psychiatric disorders: A meta-analysis.' *The Primary Care Companion to CNS Disorders, 13,* 4: PCC.10r01068.

6 Balasubramaniam, M., Telles, S., and Doraiswamy, P.M. (2012) 'Yoga on our minds: A systematic review of yoga for neuropsychiatric disorders.' *Frontiers in Psychiatry, 3,* 117.

7 McCall, T. (2007) *Yoga as Medicine.* New York: Bantam Books.

8 McCall, T. (2007) *Yoga as Medicine.* New York: Bantam Books, p.71.

9 McCall, T. (2007) *Yoga as Medicine.* New York: Bantam Books, p.72.

10 McCall, T. (2007) *Yoga as Medicine.* New York: Bantam Books.

11 Huber, C. (1988) *How You Do Anything Is How You Do Everything: A workbook.* Murphys, CA: Keep it Simple Books.

— Chapter 3 —

MORE THAN JUST A POSE

A Personal Approach to Inhabiting the Body

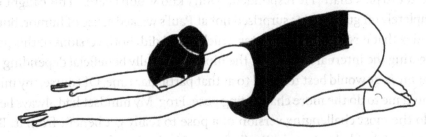

*Child gives us time to be with ourselves—whatever is showing
up—with its gentler sensations and inward focus*

Traditional yoga is primarily concerned with alignment, getting a pose to look a certain way, often to match what the teacher demonstrates. Meditation and *pranayama* are usually taught separately from the poses, either at the beginning or at the end of class. In yin yoga the breath work, physical practice, the subtle body, mindfulness, and psychological inquiry can all be done within the yoga practice, rather than as separate components. In addition, yin is much more personal than other forms of yoga. Every yin pose is a customized practice that allows a student to move into shapes that are safe and appropriate for them. In the stillness and silence of each pose, students learn how to listen to the body's cues as they come safely to their individual edge. The longer-held postures give us the time to both open up and dive deep into our inner and outer experiences.

FUNCTIONAL ALIGNMENT APPROACH

Once I discovered the power of yin for my clients, I was eager to study with some wonderful yin teachers and develop more knowledge and teaching skills. I could not wait to work with Paul Grilley and take his foundational 100-hour yin yoga training. Unlike that first time I took a yin class, I was coming into this training with a lot of yin experience. I had learned how to do all the poses, managed to increase my tolerance for discomfort, and was even able to do poses without any props. I hoped that if anyone was to evaluate my yin poses, they would rate them an A. The first night of Paul's training, he led us into a sequence and invited us to choose a variation of a pose. "You can do Frog or Wide-Knee Child or any other version you like." I asked him, "Since Frog is the more challenging version, isn't it better to pick that?" He responded, "Don't know, don't care." This caught me completely off guard. I was surprised not at Paul's wicked sense of humor, but at the idea that it really did not matter which pose I did. Both versions of this pose (targeting the internal rotators of the hips) are equally beneficial depending on what *my body* would best respond to at that particular time. Of course, my mind wanted me to do the more challenging pose, Frog. My mindset had always been to do the most challenging version of a pose to really get benefit from it. But this time, I decided to test out Paul's theory. Maybe doing less would be equally potent if my body felt safe in the pose. And that is exactly what happened. I took the shape of Wide-Knee Child pose with a blanket under my knees for support. I did not wiggle, force my mind to think about something else (like what I was going to have for dinner), or use deep breathing to get through the pose. Over time, I felt more and more spaciousness and ease in the pose.

For the next pose, Paul asked us to come into a hip opener; Sleeping Swan or its gentler sister, Deer pose. Again, while my mind wanted me to go into Pigeon, I selected Deer. This deeply settled quality began to envelop me like a warm protective blanket. Something was shifting inside me. My personal edge that tends to be hard, striving, and uncompromising softened into a kinder, gentler, softer edge.

At the end of the class, I glanced around. Students had chosen from each of the variations that were offered, using props to support various parts of the body. Each person had found a customized shape that worked for them. The energy of the room was quiet and still. This is transformational yin yoga.

Following my "ah-ha" moment with Paul Grilley, I began leading yin from a functional alignment approach. This approach recognizes that skeletal variations (the angles of the bones) will impact the exact shape the body will take in order to stress, stimulate, or move the body. Just as I observed in my yoga teacher training, each person's pose may look different, yet the target area (specific muscle group and its connective tissue) maintains the same functional intention. This intention may be to stretch, compress, or load the area to produce a yin effect. Instead of demonstrating a pose so that my students see an ideal or aesthetically pretty version of the pose, I will often lead with the more accessible variations first, calling them "Version A." For example, Stirrup pose (also known as Happy Baby pose), can be expressed by laying on one's back and drawing the feet out in front of the knees in a frog position, externally rotating the feet out toward 90 degrees; in "Version B," the feet are guided up toward the ceiling, using the hands to hold the inside or outside edges of the feet. By teaching the versions in this way, my students are more likely to select the pose that functionally works best for their body. Essentially, I am trying to remove the ego or self-judgment from the process, so they go with what works.

TO PROP OR NOT TO PROP

The use of props such as blankets, bolsters, blocks, and straps plays an important role in yin yoga as a transformational practice. While some yin yoga teachers feel that props can take away the juiciness and intensity of the pose, I have observed that props allow the body to settle more quickly once in a pose and help people to stay within a tolerable range of sensation for them. By using a sensation scale (as I suggested in Chapter 1), students can evaluate and monitor the level of sensation they are experiencing and make mindful choices. They may choose to deepen into the pose by removing the prop or to add more propping to regulate the intensity of the pose. More intensity does not equal greater success. Success is when students feel empowered to monitor, adjust, and ultimately relax into a shape that can stimulate the tissues of the body in a healthy, safe way.

Joseph came to my yoga class as a colleague from my hospital and a very private person. He was a young, athletic-looking man with earnest eyes and a quiet shy smile. He stated that he was struggling with grief/loss after recently ending his marriage. Joseph disclosed that he had never done yoga and was afraid to take a class because he was stiff, inflexible, and very self-conscious to attend a class. I suggested that he make a little "nest" for himself in the back of the room, including two blankets, a soft bolster, and an eye pillow. I invited him to follow my directions, but to mainly stay with the sensations in his body and explore a simple inquiry during the poses: "*What is happening now?*" I recognized that Joseph did not want any extra attention, as he looked

— 35 —

down at his mat and did not make eye contact with me. Instead of frequently checking in with him, I just kept a careful eye on him and did not approach him directly to make any suggestions or adjustments. At first, his awkwardness was palpable. He was looking around the room and I could see his inner critic starting to make a lot of noise in his head. I could almost hear his inner thoughts saying, "My hips don't go down like that," "I feel embarrassed," "I don't belong."

At that point, I recommended to the whole class that they might want to explore closing their eyes during the poses to be able to tune in to the sensations and breath. Joseph's practice began once he closed his eyes. He no longer worried about how he was measuring up and relied on his props to help him in many poses that require hip openers: Butterfly, Sleeping Swan, and Shoelace. At the end of class, he waited for everyone to pack up their mats, stack their blankets, and leave. When we were alone in the room, he looked at me and his eyes were soft, his face was relaxed. "That was amazing," he started. "I am going to come back next week." I asked him what he appreciated most about his practice that evening and he said, "I could really notice what was happening in my body. I felt sensations that I had never really noticed before. By staying in a pose for such a long time, I could even see how my tight areas loosened up." Joseph was sharing what so many yin students discover: yin develops and ultimately deepens our relationship with our internal experience of the body.

INTEROCEPTION AND YIN YOGA

Through the practice of yin, Joseph was able to notice sensations in his body, a state known as *interoception* awareness. According to Norman Farb and his colleagues in a *Frontiers in Psychology* article, "Interoception is the process of receiving, accessing, and appraising internal bodily signals."[1] There has been a good deal of interest in interoception over the past decade because researchers are recognizing that detecting, interpreting, and reacting to the body's signals is a complex process that can have significant effects on well-being, disease, and mental health. The more sensitive a person is to their body's signals, the greater the impact these signals may have on that person's life. Joseph's increased awareness or sensitivity to his body's sensations helped him to feel relaxed and at ease. He discovered new insights about his body which began to transform how he viewed himself.

In contrast, sometimes highly sensitive interoception can create feelings of distress and anxiety. My mother, Gloria, is a very healthy and vibrant 81-year-old woman. She prides herself on her organic whole foods-based diet and her daily exercise routine. However, my mother has interoceptive sensitivity that can cause her extreme distress. If she notices some discomfort in her elbow after doing Tai Chi, she becomes alarmed and will immediately discontinue the exercise altogether, without exploring whether it was the Tai Chi move or perhaps some pre-existing inflammation that caused the difficulty. Her hypersensitivity leads to actions (or in this case, inaction) that deprive her of healthy movement and ultimately, feelings of vitality.

Farb and colleagues describe the need for guidance in regulating the signals of the body: "Thus, interoceptive sensitivity may either contribute or detract from well-being, suggesting a need for guidance in regulating salient visceral signals."[2] While my mother tends to be a very sensitive responder to interoceptive signals, there are many of us who struggle with too little interoceptive detection. This can occur for a variety of reasons, including a high pain tolerance, use of drugs and alcohol, or trauma. In the case of trauma, men and women with history of interpersonal violence and abuse may use dissociation when they experience sensations that are painful, uncomfortable, or have certain associations with their particular trauma (e.g., smells, sounds, tastes). Dissociation creates a separation from the body, allowing the person to essentially live outside their body for a period of time. While it was originally a way to establish safety in conditions that were life-threatening, dissociation can prevent a person from responding skillfully to the signals of the body, including pleasurable experiences that come from embodied presence and awareness. New theories in the areas of psychology, biology, and neuroscience suggest that greater accuracy in interoception can help people develop an enhanced sense of safety and well-being, improved interpersonal relationships, and increased capacity for managing stress.[3, 4, 5] There is emerging support in the research that practices such as yoga and mindfulness can "support the process of interoceptive re-discovery."[6]

One of my most challenging clients, Fran, struggled with faulty interoceptive detection. Fran is a 35-year-old woman who had a long history of childhood sexual and physical abuse from age five through age 12. She developed significant trauma-related psychological distress, including panic attacks, anger outbursts, and self-harming behaviors. Her self-harm included cutting her arms, inserting items into her skin (glass, paper clips), and ingesting non-food items, including batteries. These behaviors became life-threatening, requiring several long hospitalizations to try to eliminate them.

I asked Fran to describe what she feels before, during, and after a self-harm episode. She told me that when she feels hurt, rejected, or unloved, she notices intense pain in her chest. She interprets this bodily signal with alarm and what follows is a sense of urgency to act, usually to hurt herself. This urge grows stronger and stronger and "there is nothing I can do to make it go away." The only thing she can think of is to hurt herself in some way. During the act of self-harm, she reports that "I don't feel anything," even when she is breaking skin and bleeding. This absence of feeling the sensation of pain is a sign of dissociation, as she is not able to detect the body's pain signals that are present in that moment. After the episode, she describes feeling flooded by physical and emotional pain: "All I know is that I need help now."

Fran's case highlights a complex inner relationship with what is happening in her body. At times, she displays excessive sensitivity to interoceptive cues in her body, causing her to need to act, usually in an aggressive way, when she feels pain in her body relating to emotional distress. She tries to regulate the uncomfortable response through her self-harming behavior, which then causes her to dissociate and actively ignore interoceptive cues of pain. This fluctuation between excessive interoceptive sensitivity and dissociation effectively shuts down the interoception system in the body. This can create havoc for those suffering from this predicament, like Fran, who is desperate to break the cycle of self-harm.

Yin can be an effective way to calibrate or recalibrate one's interoception system so that a person can choose to modify or simply stay and track what is happening in their body through mindful attention and skillful action. By using a pose to connect to the body, yin students can enliven their interoceptive system, training the brain to accurately detect signals and create a safe home within the body. For clients like Fran, yin yoga can be the start of a new relationship with the body and ultimately, can start the healing journey from long-standing trauma.

Fran was very reluctant to do yoga. In fact, when I met her, she was lying in a hospital bed and did not want to get up and meet me for our first session. I asked her if she would prefer to try yoga in bed and she barely nodded yes, but she did open her eyes to look at me. I had brought a bolster and asked if she would be willing to slide the bolster under her lower back so that she could take a Supported Bridge pose. Again, she nodded slightly, and I showed her where to position the bolster to support her lower back/hips and encouraged her to notice the quality of her breath and the different physical sensations she was experiencing.

I remained quiet and just sat with her as she breathed. After about ten breaths, I asked her to tell me what she noticed. She said, in a very quiet voice, "I feel my legs working, almost like they are quivering." I asked her how intense the sensations were on a scale of one to ten and she shook her head. "I don't know." I went over the yin sensation scale with her, and she took her time to slowly answer. "I guess a two, no, maybe three."

Okay! Now we were getting somewhere. She was detecting some signals in the body and was actually present and alert. I asked her if she wanted to come out of the pose and she said that she was okay. After another ten breaths, I slowly guided her out of the pose. We did a few more poses in bed this way, a Twist (reclining) and a Supported Fish. Each time, I asked her to tell me where she felt the sensations in her body, the intensity, and whether she wanted to stay in the pose or come out. By the end of the brief bedside yin yoga session, Fran told me that she liked the practice, and that it was not as hard as she thought it would be.

Fran had taken an important step during this practice to recalibrate her body's detection system. She was able to accurately detect the location of physical sensations and their intensity and was able to be attentive and present with the sensations. She did not zone out and get lost in her thoughts, nor did she try to intensify or create distress in her body. She found a place in her body where she remained connected and safe, under her own control.

YIN AND INQUIRY

The questions that I asked Fran during the yin poses were done in a very specific way. They were designed to evoke curiosity and interest in what was happening in the body. This type of questioning is called *self-inquiry*. Self-inquiry is a form of investigation, a way to unpack and go deeper into our own inner experience.

Self-inquiry always begins with a question, something that we want to know the answer to, but we don't actually know. If we already know the answer, then there is no point in doing an inquiry. We do this all the time when we berate ourselves by saying, "Why am I so stupid?" "What's wrong with me?" These are not true inquiry questions because they are done with a critical voice rather than an open, curious voice, and they cannot really be answered in any meaningful way. The two keys to self-inquiry are *not-knowing* and *openness to exploration*; what I like to call *true curiosity*. The purpose of inquiry is to go beyond the everyday discursive mind, the familiar images we have of ourselves—how we take ourselves to be. Self-inquiry can be done through a yin yoga pose, or by writing or speaking, or in a dyad with a partner. It is important to try not to direct the inquiry or have an agenda. Sometimes the answers become clear right away and sometimes they do not; this may be the doorway to more inquiry later on. Each time you practice self-inquiry, you are letting go of old patterns and ways of judging and opening up to a fresh perspective about yourself. Such an undertaking can also facilitate the creation of an accurate interoceptive system in the body, which can, in turn, create a deeper connection with one's inner and outer experiences.

Self-inquiry can be done in many types of body-based practices, including yoga. Yin yoga, in particular, is a wonderful platform for this investigation because it is slow, quiet, and spacious. Each pose, typically held for several minutes, lends itself beautifully to this type of methodical unpacking. Self-inquiry questions are designed to be asked slowly, with time to digest and process them before moving on to the next question. Trying to do self-inquiry during a Vinyasa class would be quite difficult because the body is moving quickly and there is little time to check in and deepen the experience. Yin, on the other hand, is slow. As the famous Jungian analyst Marian Woodman says, "If we could allow the pace of our meetings to slow down to the pace of our hearts, we might find genuine understanding."[7] She is essentially inviting understanding to come by moving at the soul's pace rather than the mind's rapid-fire urgency. We take our time to come into the pose, to adjust and support ourselves as needed, and then coming into a period of quiet reflection which is the foundation for self-inquiry.

Yin yoga is a personal practice designed to allow yoga students to inhabit their body within the safety of the yoga mat. Each pose teaches students how to host physical sensations and develop more accurate and sensitive interoception. Self-inquiry can assist in understanding how physical sensations in the body can impact our thoughts, feelings, and emotions with curiosity and nonjudgment. Over time, I have watched many yin students transfer these embodied practices off the yoga mat and into the world. They become more curious, open, and mindful when they are relating to others. Even more importantly, they become capacitated to host whatever is arising for themselves with more compassion and kindness.

ENDNOTES

1   Farb, N., Daubenmier, J., Price, C.J., et al. (2015) 'Interoception, contemplative practice, and health.' Frontiers in Psychology, 6, 1–26.
2   Farb, N., Daubenmier, J., Price, C.J., et al. (2015) 'Interoception, contemplative practice, and health.' Frontiers in Psychology, 6, 1–26.
3   Farb, N., Daubenmier, J., Price, C.J., et al. (2015) 'Interoception, contemplative practice, and health.' Frontiers in Psychology, 6, 1–26.

4   Craig, A.D. (2012) 'How do you feel? Interoception: The sense of the physiological condition of the body.' *Nature Reviews, 3*, 655–666.
5   Ceunen, E., Vlaeyan, J.W.S., and Van Diest, L. (2016) 'On the origin of interoception.' *Frontiers in Psychology, 7*, 1–17.
6   Farb, N., Daubenmier, J., Price, C.J., *et al.* (2015) 'Interoception, contemplative practice, and health.' *Frontiers in Psychology, 6*, 1–26.
7   Woodman, M. (2000) *Coming Home to Myself: Reflections for nurturing a woman's body and soul*. Newburyport, MA: Conari Press, p.230.

— Chapter 4 —

IMPACT OF YIN YOGA ON THE NERVOUS SYSTEM

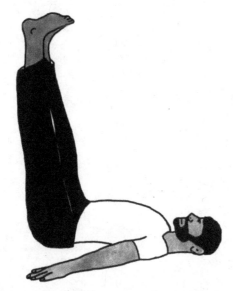

In Legs Up the Wall pose, the ground provides stability, and the wall facilitates safety which in turn supports healing

When we are in an emotional or stress-related crisis, our whole nervous system is affected, producing potentially harmful changes in the mind and body. Yin yoga can help mitigate some of these harmful changes in very simple and accessible ways. Yin sequences work directly with the nervous system in a beautiful way, using the breath and mindful attention as the primary vehicles to ease suffering. These sequences allow us to stop reacting to stress and learn how to respond to the emotional and physical signals in the body with awareness, curiosity, and compassion. There is a growing body of research on utilizing yoga practices, including breath, poses, and meditation, for nervous system regulation. This has been measured by looking at heart rate variability, neurotransmitter systems, oxygen consumption, blood pressure, and changes in brain wave activity. The findings suggest that yoga-based practices, including yin yoga, can reduce stress-related symptoms and play a significant role in the treatment of disorders that are influenced by the nervous system.[1,2,3]

When I first start teaching yin yoga to new students and clients in a therapeutic setting, I often have them complete the Perceived Stress Scale (PSS).[4] This is a ten-question Likert scale assessing the degree to which situations are perceived as stressful. As I review the questionnaires with them, many are surprised to find that their stress levels fall in the *high perceived stress* category. They start to recognize that certain situations are overwhelming, unpredictable, or uncontrollable, and how that can create high levels of stress for them. Without directly acknowledging their stress, many people are living in a constant state of psychological and physiological tension that can create or exacerbate emotional conditions such as depression and anxiety. Once the impact of stress is truly recognized, I find that people are much more willing to utilize positive coping strategies to manage stress, including yin yoga and meditation. At the end of even a few sessions, many of my students are amazed at how far reduced their stress scores are. What is particularly exciting is that the effects remain long after the session is completed.

WHAT IS STRESS?

Stress can mean many things to different people. It can be somewhat mild, like the stress we experience when we have too many commitments in a day and can't get them all done, or severe, as in cases of repeated high-impact stress events that occur when someone was abused as a child. Therefore, when people say that they are "stressed out," I don't presume to know how intense their stress may be and how it is impacting them. I find that people are more comfortable using the word "stress" rather than "I feel depressed," "I have experienced trauma," or "I have a panic disorder." The self-perception of "stress" can be a doorway into some deep inner healing once people learn tools that can help them reduce the impact of stress on their physical bodies, nervous systems, and emotions.

The relationship between stress and the body was first advanced by psychologist Walter Cannon in the 1930s. He is credited with describing "the stress response" and introducing the physical-psychological component known as *flight or fight* that occurs when a person is experiencing stress.[5]

Twenty years later, in the 1950s, Hans Selye was credited as the founder of modern stress research through his General Adaptation Syndrome theory, which spelled out the impact of stress on the nervous system through neural and hormonal processes. He described how the impact of long-term stress can result in damage to the different physiological systems in the body, including the heart, digestion, immune system, and kidneys.[6]

In the 1970s, psychologist R.S. Lazarus delineated three different kinds of psychological stress states: harm, threat, and challenge. Lazarus focused on how we appraise a situation, which he called *cognitive mediational outlook,* as a key component of whether someone experiences stress as a threat or as a challenge. He also emphasized *coping* in his stress model. "Coping shapes emotion, as it does psychological stress, by influencing the person-environment relationship and how it is appraised."[7]

Lazarus emphasized strategies to ameliorate the impact of stress. He posited that a stressful situation can be shifted into a more neutral or even benign stimulus. He described how a person can overcome psychological stress by using a series of small problem-solving steps called *problem-focused coping,* in addition to *emotion-focused coping* which involves changing the way we interpret what is happening.[8] Both problem-focused coping and emotion-focused coping are utilized in many modern cognitive-behavioral and mindfulness approaches to stress management.

In the late 1980s, A.Z. Reznick described stress as a cycle with four distinct phases: *resting, tension, response, and relief.*[9] The tension phase, either physical or psychological, can be divided into negative or positive categories. When strain is perceived as unpleasant or uncomfortable, this is considered "negative strain." On the other hand, "positive strain" occurs if the sensations or emotions are perceived as thrilling, creative, or part of overcoming a challenge. This model is helpful when understanding how the same strain can be stressful depending on the person, how they perceive the sensation, and the outcome of the activity producing the strain. For example, when I train for marathons, I have to do very long training runs. During my long runs, there are all sorts of uncomfortable sources of tension in my body and my mind. However, I perceive them as positive because they are reflecting my hard work and are part of the bigger goal. The final phase, relief, includes both the physical and psychological release from strain and stress and the return to the resting phase.

Reznick's cycle of stress is a helpful model when understanding the transformational quality of yin yoga. The sensations that occur during yin yoga have this quality that Reznick describes as *tension.* In fact, yin poses are targeting the connective tissue in such a way as to cause tension through tugging, pulling, and loading the fascia and connective tissue throughout the body. For new students, this can be a negative experience, causing a stress response or strong desire to move away from the sensations. However, over time, with careful guidance and slow acclimation to the sensations, this same tension is perceived as positive, as the outcome is now known to the student. The tension actually helps the body to find more fluidity, range of motion, comfort, and ease. This shift from *negative tension* to *positive tension* can have far-reaching effects in terms of how we respond to stress. We learn to stay longer with discomfort, to use mindfulness to track the sensations, and to use skillful methods of self-care and response rather than extreme or impulsive reactions to just get rid of the feeling we don't like. The relief phase comes much more quickly when we can meet tension skillfully and learn to fully release and return to our natural state of being. Figure 4.1 describes this positive cycle for yin yoga practice.

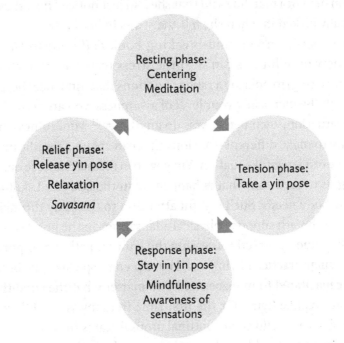

Figure 4.1 Positive stress cycle for yin yoga
(Adapted from Reznick)[10]

Once a positive stress cycle has been established using yin yoga, students begin to expand their bandwidth to meet other stressful situations off the mat as well. One of my longtime yin yoga students, Sue, shared with me that she had a fear of flying that had kept her off planes for the past decade or more. But now she wanted to visit her new grandson in Florida, which would require her to fly. She said she was not sure how the flight would go and was armed with medications, lots of books, and a good deal of fear. A few weeks later, she happily informed me that she had made the trip successfully and had been so surprised that her anxiety had been manageable. She explained that she felt the anxiety and discomfort in her body as she had expected, but she knew from her years-long yin yoga practice how to handle these feelings: by breathing, sensing into her body, and creating a warmth and friendliness toward her fear. She did not simply react to the stress by getting dysregulated, by crying, by using medications or alcohol, or by trying to push the stress away and ignore it, a strategy we often call "white knuckling it." Instead, she responded to her stress using the tools that she had honed so well with her regular yin yoga practice. This made all the difference in her experience. The most exciting part of Sue's story is that she was able to respond to stress without even consciously trying to use these tools and methods; it was instinctive after years of practicing a positive stress response on her yoga mat. She said that she had just noticed how these practices automatically kicked in when she felt the stress in her body.

In Jon Kabat-Zinn's ground-breaking book *Full Catastrophe Living*, he describes how mindfulness can shift the stress response from automatically occurring (reacting) to offering a range of options that influence the next actions (responding): "By increasing your level of awareness, you are actually changing the entire situation, even before you do anything."[11] Mindfulness gives us the opportunity to make different decisions that can create a significant change in the outcome of a stressful situation. Yin yoga can further increase our awareness by inviting us to focus on what is happening in the body and skillfully attend to what the body needs. Such skillful attention to the body through a variety of means (e.g., breath support, physical adaptations in the pose) can expedite a return to baseline by directly accessing the parasympathetic response system. Through regular practice of yin yoga, I have seen people like Sue become more and more capacitated to manage stress, no matter what the conditions—even novel situations like flying for the first time in many years. Effectively, they have been able to extend their "optimal arousal states in which emotions can be experienced as tolerable and experience can be integrated,"[12] according to Corrigan *et al.* 2011.

In 1994, Stephen Porges introduced the polyvagal theory "as an expansive brain-body model that emphasized the bidirectional communication between the brain and the body."[13] The theory was embraced by clinicians, body workers, and yoga therapists because it provided a missing link in understanding trauma and its impact on the nervous system and the perception of safety. Polyvagal theory focuses on the evolutionary link between the vagus nerve and the autonomic nervous system. Porges' theory posits that there are three distinct "neural platforms" that are the underpinning for the overall autonomic nervous system and directly influence perceptions, emotions, and behaviors. The oldest and most primitive branch of the vagus nerve (named the dorsal vagal complex or DVC) is responsible for the immobilization or shutdown of an organism in response to the detection of danger, often associated with the "freeze" response. The target of this response is the visceral organs. The next system in evolutionary development is the sympathetic nervous system (SNS). This system's primary function is to mobilize some type of action, the familiar "fight or flight" behavior seen in response to danger. From an evolutionary development perspective, the most recently developed neural platform, the ventral vagal complex (VVC), exists only in mammals. The VVC utilizes the "ventral" branch of the parasympathetic nervous system and is linked to cranial nerves that control the muscles of the head, face, middle ear, pharynx, bronchi, and heart. Porges calls this platform the "social engagement system" because it is the system that helps orient us toward human connection and engagement in prosocial behaviors, and ultimately toward a feeling of safety.[14, 15, 16]

According to Porges, this perception of safety—or lack of it—is called *neuroception*,[17] the "subconscious detection of safety or danger in the environment" through vagal sensory inputs.[18] What is important about this concept of neuroception is that our responses to stress are often happening prior to the higher brain centers becoming aware of what is going on. In other words, whether we feel safe or feel threatened is a perception that often happens outside of our conscious awareness, yet our bodies are responding. Yin yoga and other mind-body practices can help support a more accurate interpretation of mind, body, and environmental stimuli by consciously and nonjudgmentally investigating such stimuli as they are happening in the present moment. This "reappraisal of stimuli" through present-moment awareness of physical sensations and emotions can help regulate the nervous system and activate the VVC.[19, 20, 21]

When the VVC is engaged, a person has greater capacity to regulate emotions and more flexibility in how to respond to stress. There is a sense of safety and security. Furthermore, this system, when functioning optimally, can foster compassion and love through human engagement, which is key to a sense of happiness and stability in a person's mental health. Therefore, our yin yoga and mindfulness methods can help us exercise or "practice" shaping our nervous system regulation to benefit our physical and mental health.[22, 23, 24]

A practical model that integrates the impacts of stress on the nervous system that we have been exploring is called the *window of tolerance*.[25] As a psychologist, I find this model very helpful in understanding the effects of stress, especially with my clients who have experienced trauma. The window of tolerance model, which describes the autonomic arousal response to stress, was developed by the psychiatrist Dan Siegel who specializes in the field of interpersonal neurobiology to transform psychological conditions.[26, 27]

Siegel's model suggests that there is a range of optimal functioning, a "window," in which a person can effectively cope with emotions, integrate experiences, and interact with others in the world. Essentially, this window allows people to both think and feel to cope effectively even when they are in the midst of stressful situations. This window is situated in between the more extreme states of sympathetic-driven nervous system hyperarousal (fight or flight, reactive, flooded) and parasympathetic-driven nervous system hypoarousal (dissociation/numbing/hopelessness). Pat Ogden and other trauma experts have specifically focused on how trauma can alter the nervous system so that the window of tolerance effectively shrinks and there is less and less capacity to cope with stressors, leaving people either in a chronically hyperaroused or hypoaroused state (or sometimes both).[28, 29]

Yin yoga can help people to develop self-regulation skills that can positively influence the window of tolerance, increasing their capacity to manage stress and their self-perception that they have this capacity. As I will share in the story to follow, with repeated practice these skills often generalize to our daily lives, creating resilience.

Emma was referred to me for yoga therapy after she experienced a major behavioral episode in a general yoga class. She became extremely dysregulated in the class, talking loudly, yelling at the teacher when she could not understand how to do a pose, and then began crying loudly. The teacher kindly went over and spoke to her and invited her to take a Child's pose, *Savasana*, or simply sit quietly. Emma was embarrassed and left the room but did stay in the studio until the class was finished to talk with the teacher. She reported that she was having flashbacks in the middle of the class, remembering when her mother was verbally and physically abusive to her when she did not do her chores the way she was supposed to or when she tried to stand up for herself. Emma was currently in psychiatric care, with both a psychiatrist and a counselor working together to help her with her distress. They had recommended yoga to her, which many mental health professionals do because it can be so beneficial. However, a general yoga class for someone who has trauma and, effectively, a relatively small window of tolerance, can actually create more stress. As it did for Emma, going to a general yoga class can potentially leave the person feeling even worse than when they started, by bringing up unresolved trauma and feelings of negative self-worth.

The wise yoga teacher suggested that Emma met with me to do some yoga therapy so that she could explore the benefits of yoga in a supported and individualized (and safer) manner, and Emma agreed.

When I met with Emma for the first time, I was struck by how anxious and aroused she appeared. Emma is a tall, thin, striking woman in her mid-50s with silver-gray hair and beautiful blue eyes. She had poor eye contact, displayed rapid speech, and appeared anxious. Emma reported that she had practiced yoga on and off for the last 20 years and had found it helpful in the past. However, recently, yoga had been triggering when she was around other people in a class setting. She described that whenever she thought that she was doing something wrong and was going to be singled out, she started to get anxious and upset.

I asked Emma to let her mind float back to the yoga class last week when she was dysregulated. I gently questioned her: "What was first thing you noticed when you became upset?" She stated that it was a series of negative thoughts that first triggered her. She described the thoughts which came rapid-fire, one after the other: "I can't see what the teacher is doing. I am doing it wrong. I am going to get in trouble." I asked her to describe what happened next. "Then, I just started panicking. I stopped thinking and I felt desperate. I needed help and I could not get it." I asked her to describe where she felt it in her body. "My heart is pounding, my vision is blurry, and I feel like I am going to faint. I have to get out of here."

Emma was describing a classic presentation of nervous system hyper-arousal, triggered by her long trauma history. Her cognitive appraisal, "I am going to get in trouble," sent power messages to her body that she needed to *do something*. In this case, her body was responding to a perceived threat, and she was not able to think or talk her way out of the situation. As she shared and reflected on her experience, she became more and more agitated, the story itself seeming to trigger another hyperarousal episode.

I invited Emma to try an experiment with me, if she was willing. I had her place her legs up on the wall in an inversion. An inversion pose can often support relaxation for the nervous system through a physiological response to the legs resting above the heart. I then asked her to report what she was noticing. She said that her heart was pounding, her legs felt shaky and weak as they rested against the wall. I continued to ask her to label her experiences and she went on to report that "my palms are sweaty, my stomach feels tight and clenched, and I feel cold." I continued to ask her to report for the next several minutes, just having her meet her experiences directly and name them while I held the space, occasionally reflecting back what she was saying, or simply saying, "Tell me more."

Her voice became quieter and softer after about ten minutes of this practice. There were longer spaces where she was just breathing and sensing in the body. I asked her to just continue to notice whatever signals her body wanted to share. Her eyes were now closed, and breathing was slow and steady. I had her lower her legs and rest on her back for a few moments and then come back to a seated position. I asked her to reflect on how that practice was for her. She shared that at first, she wanted to get up and bolt. The urge to flee was strong. However, as she started naming her body sensations, she noticed that the sensations began to decrease in their intensity. "I felt like I could stay for a little while longer and I wasn't going to die." She reported that after a while, she felt a warm relaxation take over, as if her body was completely wrung out like a sponge and all she wanted to do was rest and relax. She said that it was a pleasant experience and she wanted to stay like that for a while. She said that she was surprised that ten minutes had gone by, as she felt like it was just a minute or two that had passed.

Emma was now comfortably within her window of tolerance. I talked with her about using the inversion pose as a foundation yin yoga practice that she could do each day, learning how to notice, label, and observe different sensations and emotions. She could stay in the pose for as long or as little as she needed to. The key was for her to identify her experiences and stay with them in a safe place where she felt enough physical and emotional support to be able to withstand the experience. The idea for a daily practice using a yin pose along with a cognitive label was to help Emma skillfully increase her window of tolerance using interoceptive cues and a grounding pose. The yin window of tolerance can be a helpful tool to monitor one's response to the pose. If someone has become sympathetically aroused, they can use techniques such as labeling and noting, mindfulness, and breath as anchors to return to their window. Each time they are able to successfully attune to their experience and find relief, much as Emma did, their capacity to cope with stress increases, as well as building confidence in their own ability to work through challenges. This can translate off the yoga mat into everyday life, as they can feel a sense of control around managing episodes of hyper- (or hypo-) arousal.

ENDNOTES

1   Streeter, C., Gerbarg, P., Saper, R., Ciraulo, D., and Brown, R. (2012) 'Effects of yoga on the autonomic nervous system, gamma-aminobutyric-acid, and allostasis in epilepsy, depression, and post-traumatic stress disorder.' *Medical Hypotheses, 78*, 5, 571–579.

2   Jerath, R., Edry, J., Barnes, V., and Jerath, V. (2006) 'Physiology of long pranayamic breathing: Neural respiratory elements may provide a mechanism that explains how slow deep breathing shifts the autonomic nervous system.' *Medical Hypotheses, 67*, 3, 566–571.

3   Brown, R., Gerbarg, P., and Muench, F. (2013) 'Breathing practices for the treatment of psychiatric and stress-related medical conditions.' *Psychiatric Clinics of North America, 36*, 1, 121–140.

4   Cohen, S., Kamarck, T., and Mermelstein, R. (1983) 'A global measure of perceived stress.' *Journal of Health and Social Behavior, 24*, 386–396.

5   Rom, O., and Reznick, A. (2016) 'The stress reaction: A historical perspective.' *Advances in Experimental Medicine and Biology, 20*, 1–4.

6   Lazarus, R.S. (1993) 'From psychological stress to the emotions: A history of changing outlooks.' *Annual Review of Psychology, 44*, 1–21.

7   Lazarus, R.S. (1993) 'From psychological stress to the emotions: A history of changing outlooks.' *Annual Review of Psychology, 44*, 1–21.

8   Lazarus, R.S. (1993) 'From psychological stress to the emotions: A history of changing outlooks.' *Annual Review of Psychology, 44*, 1–21.

9   Reznick, A.Z. (1989) 'The cycle of stress: A circular model for the psychobiological response to strain and stress.' *Medical Hypotheses, 30*, 217–222.

10   Reznick, A.Z. (1989) 'The cycle of stress: A circular model for the psychobiological response to strain and stress.' *Medical Hypotheses, 30*, 217–222.

11   Kabat-Zinn, J. (2013) *Full Catastrophe Living: Using the wisdom of your body and mind to face stress, pain, and illness.* New York: Bantam Books, p.288.

12   Corrigan, F., Fisher, J., and Nutt, D. (2011) 'Autonomic dysregulation and the Window of Tolerance model of the effects of complex emotional trauma.' *Journal of Psychopharmacology, 25*, 1, 17–25.

13   Porges, S. (2003) 'The polyvagal theory: Phylogenetic contributions to social behavior.' *Physiology & Behavior, 79*, 3, 503–513.

14   Porges, S. (2003) 'The polyvagal theory: Phylogenetic contributions to social behavior.' *Physiology & Behavior, 79*, 3, 503–513.

15   Porges, S. (2011) *The Polyvagal Theory: Neurophysiological foundations of emotions, attachment, communication, and self-regulation.* New York: W.W. Norton.

16   Sullivan, M., Erb, M., Schmalzl, L., Moonaz, S., Taylor, J., and Porges, S. (2018) 'Yoga therapy and polyvagal theory: The convergence of traditional wisdom and contemporary neuroscience for self-regulation and resilience.' *Frontiers in Human Neuroscience*, 27 February.

17   Porges, S. (2003) 'The polyvagal theory: Phylogenetic contributions to social behavior.' *Physiology & Behavior, 79*, 3, 503–513.

18   Sullivan, M., Erb, M., Schmalzl, L., Moonaz, S., Taylor, J., and Porges, S. (2018) 'Yoga therapy and polyvagal theory: The convergence of traditional wisdom and contemporary neuroscience for self-regulation and resilience.' *Frontiers in Human Neuroscience.* doi: 10.3389/fnhum.2018.00067.

19   Porges, S. (2003) 'The polyvagal theory: Phylogenetic contributions to social behavior.' *Physiology & Behavior, 79*, 3, 503–513.

20   Porges, S. (2011) *The Polyvagal Theory: Neurophysiological foundations of emotions, attachment, communication, and self-regulation.* New York: W.W. Norton.

21   Sullivan, M., Erb, M., Schmalzl, L., Moonaz, S., Taylor, J., and Porges, S. (2018) 'Yoga therapy and polyvagal theory: The convergence of traditional wisdom and contemporary neuroscience for self-regulation and resilience.' *Frontiers in Human Neuroscience*, 27 February.

22 Porges, S. (2003) 'The polyvagal theory: Phylogenetic contributions to social behavior.' *Physiology & Behavior, 79*, 3, 503–513.

23 Porges, S. (2011) *The Polyvagal Theory: Neurophysiological foundations of emotions, attachment, communication, and self-regulation.* New York: W.W. Norton.

24 Sullivan, M., Erb, M., Schmalzl, L., Moonaz, S., Taylor, J., and Porges, S. (2018) 'Yoga therapy and polyvagal theory: The convergence of traditional wisdom and contemporary neuroscience for self-regulation and resilience.' *Frontiers in Human Neuroscience.* doi: 10.3389/fnhum.2018.00067.

25 Siegel, D.J. (2012) *The Developing Mind: How relationships and the brain interact to shape who we are* (2nd ed.). New York: Guilford Press.

26 Corrigan, F., Fisher, J., and Nutt, D. (2011) 'Autonomic dysregulation and the Window of Tolerance model of the effects of complex emotional trauma.' *Journal of Psychopharmacology, 25*, 1, 17–25.

27 Siegel, D.J. (2012) *The Developing Mind: How relationships and the brain interact to shape who we are* (2nd ed.). New York: Guilford Press.

28 Corrigan, F., Fisher, J., and Nutt, D. (2011) 'Autonomic dysregulation and the Window of Tolerance model of the effects of complex emotional trauma.' *Journal of Psychopharmacology, 25*, 1, 17–25.

29 Ogden, P., Minton, K., and Pain, C. (2006) *Trauma and the Body: A sensorimotor approach to psychotherapy* (Norton Series on Interpersonal Neurobiology). New York: W.W. Norton.

Chapter 5

IMPACT OF YIN YOGA ON EMOTIONS

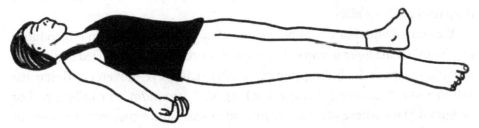

*In Savasana, we can simply observe the ever-changing flow
of breath, sensations, emotions, and thoughts*

Many of the clients I work with in inpatient settings struggle with negative emotions. Some of these are related to their specific mental health symptoms (depression, anxiety, paranoia), while others are due in part to the impact of long-term institutionalization. When the treatment, in this case being in a locked mental health facility, can either cause additional psychiatric symptoms to emerge or a current condition to worsen, this is called an *iatrogenic effect*.

I was asked to run a mindful yoga group on a long-term unit in the forensic building on the hospital campus. This unit housed clients who had been at the hospital for many years or were facing long commitment terms by order of the criminal justice system. The group was voluntary, and I was not sure if anyone would actually show up. Why would they want to do yoga? Would they think it was ridiculous to try to work on inner peace and relaxation while living in a virtual prison? To my surprise, six men showed up for the first class. They were a diverse group: Black, white, and Hispanic, ranging in age from 21 to 50. We went around and introduced ourselves. I asked the men to share something they hoped to get out of the class. Most of them answered that they wanted to feel more relaxed and calmer. One man said he liked exercise and thought it would help him feel more fit. One man, the youngest in the group, said that he was not sure, but he had always enjoyed meditation and spirituality before his psychiatric illness took over.

We started the group by going over the basics just like I do every beginner group. We reviewed safety, trusting/listening to the body, and basic components of a yoga class. I had them complete a pre-test called the "Subjective Units of Distress Scale" or SUDS. It is a simple Likert scale asking them to rank how much distress they are in from zero to ten, with zero reflecting no stress and ten indicating extreme distress. Each man filled out the brief form and the average was between five and six. We were in a small room with fluorescent lights and plastic green chairs. Not exactly the most therapeutic space, but we made do. The men rolled out their mats and I began with a guided meditation called yoga *nidra,* which can produce states between sleep and wakefulness where deep healing takes place.

We started with body sensing and breath awareness, and then I introduced an idea called the *inner resource.* The inner resource has been utilized in different somatic practices, including somatic experiencing, eye movement desensitization and reprocessing therapy (EMDR), and yoga *nidra.*[1] It can be a real or imagined place where one feels calm and at ease, and experiences a sense of well-being. It is often a nature image like the ocean or mountains, or it can be a person or beloved pet, symbol, or spiritual guide. It can also be a place in the body where one feels warm and relaxed. The inner resource can be used during meditation, as part of a yin yoga practice, or any time during the day when a person might be overwhelmed by emotions, thoughts, or situations.

For my clients, I thought it would be very important to spend time cultivating their inner resources, given the setting we were in and their psychiatric conditions, which often created feelings of overwhelm. I had them go around and share what their inner resource was: "The ocean," "my backyard," "I don't know," "my bedroom," no response, and "my daughter." I invited them to imagine their inner resource using all their senses to help make the image vibrant and clear.

After meditation, we did some warm-ups and then I offered only one simple yin pose: legs up on the heavy plastic chairs. We moved our mats close to the chairs and I showed them how they could rest their legs up on the chair in this inversion. We spent five minutes like this, breathing and returning to the inner resource. After the class, I asked the men to complete their SUDS scale again. Each of them shared their ratings with the rest of the group. The average score had dropped to two points. While this was not a huge reduction, it was still quite significant for this group of clients, who had been in treatment for many months or years with no improvement. We ended the group bowing to each other and saying, "namaste." The men rolled up their mats. There were loud noises outside the room. Voices calling, "dining room," and the jostling of clients and keys jangling.

One man stayed back to talk to me. He was the youngest in the group, just 21 years old. He had been in the hospital for about six months. He said to me, "I did not know that I could feel calm in this place, but I did today. I did not know that I could find beauty again in here, but I did." He shared that his inner resource was the backyard of his home, which overlooked a meadow and rolling hills. Then he said something that was so touching that I can still remember to this day how it opened my heart. He said, "I can go to this place anytime now, and I know I will be okay."

THE ROLE OF EMOTIONS

When a person is experiencing a greater proportion of negative emotions to positive emotions, we may consider this *emotional imbalance.* However, it is not just about the ratio of negative to positive feelings that creates this sense of imbalance. Emotional imbalance can develop according to how we relate or don't relate to our emotions. For example, if we can respond to difficult emotions in a skillful manner, we become more resilient, leading to a sense of balance and well-being. However, if we meet our difficult emotions with reactivity, blame, and shame, we only intensify the emotional imbalance in our inner world, leaving us vulnerable to depression, anxiety, and other mental health conditions.

One of the challenges in achieving emotional balance is that we are biologically wired to look for the negative as part of our survival as a species. Rick Hanson, author of *Buddha's Brain* and *Hardwiring Happiness,*[2,3] calls this hardwiring "negativity bias." He describes how this bias developed over the course of evolution with the human brain learning how to scan for potential dangers, remembering threats that leave all humans vulnerable to a sense of discomfort and separation. He explains that "negative stimuli are perceived more rapidly and easily than positive stimuli. We recognize angry faces more quickly than happy ones; in fact, the brain will react even without your conscious awareness when another person's face is angry."[4] Further, Hanson describes how "Bad (painful, upsetting) experiences routinely overpower good (pleasurable, comforting) ones."[5] As a result, it takes many more positive emotions to balance negative ones. The ratio of positive to negative emotions might need to be as much as three to one or even higher for a person to experience emotional balance. It is not just the event itself, but how it can impact the brain, which in turn can strengthen the negative effect. The negativity bias impacts the sympathetic nervous system in the brain, particularly the amygdala, hypothalamus, and hippocampus. This can become a vicious cycle over time, with increased sensitivity and reactivity to the negative.[6] Carla Shatz, an American neurobiologist, described this phenomenon that takes place in the brain as "cells that fire together, wire together."[7] In other words, a pattern in the brain develops between an action and a negative emotional or physical response, which in turn strengthens the likelihood of repeating the same response again the next time one encounters a similar situation. For example, if a person becomes anxious before giving a speech, they might have a racing heart, sweaty palms, and a dry mouth. If they don't utilize any coping skills in the face of this reaction, the next time they go up to speak, they will often have a similar or even more intense reaction due to the patterning that has developed, even from a single previous event. Many of us are actually strengthening this tendency to experience negative emotions (albeit unintentionally) despite our great desire to feel happy. I think about this a lot when I consider how much my clients are bothered by a perceived slight or an apparently small stressor. It is not the stressor itself, but the pattern that gets activated, which can elicit a strong negative reaction from a seemingly insignificant event.

But it's not all doom and gloom. Using this same principle of patterns that can activate neural networks in the brain, neuroscience researchers are exploring how we can also learn how *to practice* experiencing more *positive* emotions.

POSITIVE PSYCHOLOGY

The field of positive psychology has become extremely popular over the last two decades. Martin Seligman describes positive psychology as the "scientific study of the strengths that enable individuals and communities to thrive. The field is founded on the belief that people want to lead meaningful and fulfilling lives, to cultivate what is best within themselves, and to enhance their experiences of love, work, and play."[8]

In this model, positive emotions play an important role in both the development and the maintenance of well-being. Certain positive emotions, including joy, interest, contentment, pride, and love, have been linked to resilience and the development of psychological resources. Barbara Fredrickson's *broaden-and-build theory* describes how "positive emotions are vehicles for individual growth and social connection: by building people's personal and social resources, positive emotions transform people for the better, giving them better lives in the future."[9] Further, positive emotions have been demonstrated to help successfully regulate negative emotional experiences, which in turn can help to mitigate the physical and psychological toll of stress.[10]

Yoga can play an important role in fostering positive emotions. It has been found to increase positive emotions, including life satisfaction and emotional well-being, and to decrease negative emotions, such as anxiety, distress, and perceived stress, in several studies on breast cancer survivors.[11, 12, 13] Yoga has been shown to help with body image, increased body awareness, and decreased self-objectification for women.[14] A 2005 study (the only one of its kind so far) on the effects of yoga on mood in an inpatient psychiatric setting showed that clients participating in a weekly yoga class experienced significant improvement in negative emotions, including anxiety, depression, anger, fatigue, and confusion.[15] This study looked at gentle stretching and strengthening from the Mindfulness-Based Stress Reduction program, which includes a solid, basic introduction to yoga. This study is especially exciting to me in that it reveals how yoga can impact people with serious mental health issues, not just the "worried well" who show up in my drop-in classes at the yoga studio.

Finally, positive emotions can be cultivated in yoga by utilizing ancient and potent practices like loving awareness and compassion meditations. By establishing opportunities to "practice" positive emotions, yoga can help to promote a sense of calm and well-being. Yin yoga allows many opportunities for these practices as each pose provides an opportunity to reinforce positive emotions, including loving awareness, compassion, forgiveness, and many others, during the longer-held shapes. The yoga teacher or yoga therapist can guide the student into a pose and then utilize specific meditations that can help to create new patterns of well-being. For example, I will guide a student into a yin pose and then offer a meditation practice focused around opening up to positive emotions. I might ask them to recall a time where they felt safe, happy, and protected and notice where they feel that in the body. Here, I am beginning to help them connect positive emotions with felt sensations in the body, all while staying present and alert. By creating this link with emotions and the body, helping students to remain curious and open, and enhancing positive emotions through guided reflections, yin yoga can help individuals to create healthier neural network patterns in the brain.

EUDAEMONIA AND WELL-BEING

Happiness, joy, and other positive emotions are often associated with higher life satisfaction, subjective well-being, and low negative affect.[16] Physical activity, including various types of yoga, has been shown to increase a temporary sense of pleasure and well-being while the activity is being done. In addition, yoga can also enhance a more ongoing state of happiness called *eudaemonic well-being*. Eudaemonia is associated with human potential, growth, and finding meaning in life. One of my yoga therapy colleagues, researcher Marlysa Sullivan, recounts how this notion of eudaemonic well-being can be traced back to Aristotle, who described eudaemonia as an enduring rather than a transient form of happiness.[17] Sullivan explains that yoga can be a vehicle of enhancing eudaemonic well-being: "The ethical practices of yoga, such as virtue ethics, are meant to be a consistent and disciplined practice to overcome the obstacles of the mind and emotions for the alleviation of suffering and connection to the experience of awareness."[18]

Yoga practices that investigate one's personal ethics and moral concerns by using traditional yoga philosophy can be part of inquiry both on and off the yoga mat. According to traditional yoga philosophy, the *yamas* and *niyamas* are ethical guidelines to support a fulfilling spiritual life. The *yamas* (translated as "restraints") and *niyamas* (translated as "observances") are laid out as part of the first two limbs of the Eightfold Path written by Patanjali in the *Yoga Sutras* (translated as "scriptures"). The *Yoga Sutras* are considered one of the authoritative texts on yoga and the spiritual journey. They form a type of moral code of conduct that promotes introspection and mindful interaction with other people and the world at large. Deborah Adele's book *The Yamas and Niyamas*[19] is a great resource for more information on these classical yoga teachings, along with Michael's Stone's book *The Inner Tradition of Yoga*[20] and Bhava Ram's book *The Eight Limbs of Yoga*.[21] One of the *yamas*, called *ahimsa*, is translated as "non-harming" or "having compassion for all beings." In the *Yoga Sutras*, Patanjali describes in Sutra 2.35: "Being firmly grounded in nonviolence creates an atmosphere in which others can let go of their hostility."[22] This passage invites yoga practitioners to mindfully attend to their own bodies and minds in a compassionate and loving way, so that they are able to relate to others in a friendlier manner. This is the basis for our modern understanding of effective interpersonal communication and can open the door to meeting others in a much more heartfelt and open way.

J.A. Smith and colleagues, in an article titled "Is there more to yoga than exercise?", found that an integrated yoga practice, including the ethical practices of yoga (*yamas* and *niyamas*), had a greater effect on anxiety-related symptoms and salivary cortisol than physical postures (*asana*) alone.[23] Other researchers have found that the use of ethical practices in yoga can strengthen one's relationship to oneself through mindfulness and self-compassion, as well as one's relationships to others through feelings of compassion and connection.[24, 25, 26]

The social connection aspect of yoga has important implications for happiness and overall health. When people have close personal relationships, they report higher levels of well-being, emotional health, and happiness.[27] Yoga can help people feel less socially isolated and enhance a sense of belonging and connection that may lead to a deeper spiritual connection.[28] This is especially important for populations at risk for depression, isolation, and loneliness, including people who live with mental health conditions, traumatic brain injury, the elderly, and those going through interpersonal difficulties, including divorce and abuse. In teaching people with mental health conditions, the sense of belonging that occurs after even one yoga class has been gratifying to witness. After yoga practice, I have seen people's whole body transformed from guarded, withdrawn, and downcast to alive and bright and connected.

INNER RESOURCE/SAFE PLACE

There are particular practices in yoga that can further enhance this sense of well-being that have been established over the past decade. One method that I have been utilizing for my clients is the use of an *inner resource*. As I described in the example at the beginning of this chapter, the inner resource is an important part of trauma-based therapies, including Integrative Restoration (or iRest). This is a type of yoga *nidra*, a guided meditation based on yoga philosophy and psychology to help promote a sense of deep relaxation, well-being and ease. The practice of iRest, developed by Richard Miller and his team, has been used with many at-risk populations, including veterans, active military personnel, the homeless, and those with traumatic brain injury.[29]

I often include the inner resource practice in both group and individual yin classes because it is so helpful for many of my clients who are feeling fearful or depressed, or have experienced significant trauma. It can be especially helpful in the beginning of a session or practice when people are at their most vulnerable and afraid. The inner resource tool is designed to help people access a basic sense of security and well-being within themselves. It can be used proactively to establish a sense of grounding and stability at the beginning of a practice; people can also return to it as an emotion regulation tool during a practice, especially if they are overwhelmed by an emotion, sensation, or memory. People can utilize their inner resources for as long as they need to, and either return to practice or allow this to become their practice. This tool can help people learn how to draw upon their own inner strength and attune to their basic needs whenever their emotional state calls for it. Over time, people who utilize the inner resource tool find more and more opportunities for stability within themselves and learn that it is always present, even with the up-and-down challenges of life. This sense of stability can promote improved mental health, better relationships, and a sense of eudaemonic well-being.

Similar to the inner resource, the idea of a *safe place* has been utilized in different psychology models to treat trauma. Eye movement desensitization and reprocessing therapy (EMDR), developed by Francine Shapiro, describes the safe place as an "emotional oasis" that can be used as a "personal refuge" during some of the more challenging phases of processing trauma.[30] Both the inner resource and the safe place allow clients to find their own inner strength to manage anxiety, rather than looking for outside help. This can be empowering and part of increasing resilience across a lifetime. The safe place can be used as part of yin yoga and meditation practice. I often include it in the opening meditation and then provide an opportunity throughout the practice to return to the safe place within poses and at the end in *Savasana*.

INTENTION

The powerful practices described thus far in this chapter—yoga, meditation, ethical inquiry, and inner resource/safe place—can be enhanced even further by generating a specific *intention* for the practices themselves.

In his groundbreaking book *Full Catastrophe Living,* Jon Kabat-Zinn describes mindfulness as "paying attention in a particular way: on purpose, in the present moment, and nonjudgmentally."[31] He goes on to say that "your intentions set the stage for what is possible. They remind you from moment to moment of why you are practicing in the first place."[32] Shapiro and Carlson also describe how "intention is fundamental to mindfulness practice." They explain how important it is to be clear about one's intentions and to reflect on whether these are "wholesome or unwholesome, for the benefit or harm of self and others."[33] D.H. Shapiro's study in 1992 highlighted how the intentions of meditation practitioners shifted as they practiced over time from symptom relief to self-exploration to eventually helping others: "For individuals who continue to meditate, expectations and effects shift overall along a self-regulation, self-exploration, self-liberation/compassionate service continuum."[34] Similar results were replicated with cancer clients who began practicing meditation at first with the intention of stress reduction and then found that their practice evolved over time to focus on personal growth and spirituality.[35]

Richard Miller describes how intentions "represent powerful internal statements that help you fulfill your heartfelt mission. Like a compass, intentions keep you on course so that you can accomplish your heartfelt mission. Like the banks of a river, your intentions keep you flowing in the right direction."[36]

When I am leading a yin class or individual yin yoga therapy session, I invite clients to consider what their intention is for the pose, for the entire practice, for their day, and for their deepest desire for well-being. I guide people to base their intentions in the here and now. For example, instead of saying, "I hope I will feel less anxious," they might say, "I am relaxed and at ease." Many of my clients are surprised at how potent an intention set in the present moment can be for supporting their practice and their healing journey. It gives them an opportunity to *practice* experiencing positive emotions, as described earlier in this chapter with Rick Hanson's work. In yin yoga, this intention can be strengthened throughout the practice with repeated inquiry from physical shape to physical shape and throughout an entire yin sequence.

ENERGY AND EMOTIONAL BALANCE

Yoga has clearly been shown to impact mood positively and create an increased sense of emotional balance. Yin yoga is unique in that emphasizes *the flow of energy* through the body which can impact emotions and overall mental health. This understanding of energy or *Qi* in the body comes from Traditional Chinese Medicine (TCM). TCM has been practiced in China for over 2000 years, including the use of acupuncture and herbs, and the precise mapping of the body for meridians or energetic highways and acupuncture points. An in-depth exploration of TCM and the meridians are beyond the scope of this book, so I will primarily focus on the meridians as they apply to yin yoga.

There are many wonderful resources for those who are interested in learning more about TCM, including the classic text, *The Web That Has No Weaver* by Ted Kaptchuk,[37] *Between Heaven and Earth* by Harriet Beinfield and Efrem Korngold,[38] *Insight Yoga* by Sarah Powers,[39] and *Wood Becomes Water: Chinese Medicine in Everyday Life* by Gail Reichstein.[40]

This idea that yin yoga can influence the flow of energy comes from many masters, including Dr. Hiroshi Motoyama, Paul Grilley, and Sarah Powers.[41] By understanding key principles from TCM, these masters have discovered that yin yoga (through the pressurizing and tugging and pulling along different parts in the body) influences the flow of energy through specific meridians. This can have a positive impact on the body, emotions, and overall sense of well-being, especially when there are imbalances in the *Qi* flow within meridians. Yin yoga and other TCM practices, including acupuncture, herbs, and meditation, can help to rebalance deficient or depleted *Qi*.

The meridians are associated with key organs that pass through them. There are 14 major meridians in the body according to TCM. In yin yoga, we typically work with the six organ/meridian pairs located in the lower body. These include the Kidney/Urinary Bladder (UB) organ pair, Liver/Gallbladder pair, Spleen/Stomach organ pair, Lung/Large Intestine pair, and Heart/Small Intestine pair. There are both yin and yang organs that share specific meridian pathways, tissues, muscles, and energetic functions; the meridians function independently and are also in relationship with each other. The yin organs are responsible for the purifying substances and the yang organs are responsible for elimination of the "impure" substances. When organ pairs are in balance, we typically feel healthy, vibrant, and able to think clearly. When organ pairs are out of balance, we may feel illness or dis-ease, or have difficulty thinking.

TCM practitioners, including acupuncturists, are able to utilize specific treatments targeting meridians that are depleted or out of balance. For example, the Kidney organ/meridian pair and the Urinary Bladder organ/meridian pair are in direct relationship with one another. There are distinct physical, mental, energetic, and emotional qualities that are related to the Kidney/Urinary Bladder organ pair. The Kidneys, the yin organ, governs the bodily fluids and opens up into the Bladder, the yang organ, which eliminates impure or undigested food, fluids, and waste. Together they are responsible for storing vital energy for the entire body.[42, 43, 44] Mental qualities associated with this organ pair include memory, initiation, and motivation. Fear and anxiety can occur on an emotional level when this organ pair are out of balance. Similar to acupuncture treatments, people who work with a series of poses that move energy through the Kidney/UB meridians may experience a release of anxiety or fear and an increase of self-compassion, sometimes days after the practice.[45]

In my yin yoga classes, in addition to targeting the specific meridians through a sequence of poses, I will often provide specific inquiry questions to explore during these poses with the goal of creating a sense of emotional equilibrium in the body. With the Kidney/UB meridian sequence, students might explore issues related to fear or anxiety. Table 5.1 provides some general descriptions of the organ pairs and yin practices that can be utilized during such a practice. I would highly recommend Sarah Powers' book *Insight Yoga*,[46] along with the work of yin teacher and acupuncturist Josh Summer,[47] for more in-depth exploration of the meridians and yin yoga.

Table 5.1 Meridians and yin yoga

Organ pair (yin/ yang organs)	Physical	Emotional	Energetic	Mental	Yin pose (prototypes)	Yin inquiry
Kidney/Urinary Bladder	Storehouse of vital essence (Jing) and governs the hormones, health of bones, reproduction, and fluid circulation	Flexibility, openness, adaptability, and wisdom	Rules the health of the lower back, reproductive organs, lower intestinal system, and fluid system including joint lubrication	Short-term memory, mental focus, initiation, enthusiasm, limbic system functioning including controlling and regulating emotions	Forward folds (Butterfly/ Dragonfly) Backbends (Seal/Sphinx)	Recall a time when you felt anxious or fearful. Notice where you experience this in the body. Utilize the breath to experience a sense of stability and calmness even if anxiety is present.
Liver/Gall Bladder	Coordinates and regulates the movement of Qi; storehouse of blood, prevents disease, detoxifies toxic substances	Emotional balance, compassion, ability to regulate emotions skillfully	Responsible for overall healthy flow of energy, sense of balance and harmony	Discernment, planning and follow-through, creativity, and ability to change and adapt	Inner leg (Wide-Knee Child) Outer hip (Sleeping Swan)	Bring to mind a situation when you felt anger/frustration/ irritability. Notice where you experience this in the body. Instead of pushing away or resisting, stay open to the flow of energy moving through you and acknowledge your feelings are important.
Heart/Small Intestine	Governs the blood and circulatory system and generates energy	Love, joy, peace, and connection	Sense of aliveness and vitality	Mental clarity, insightfulness, helpfulness, and thoughtfulness	Inner lines of arms (Reclining twist with arm) Heart-openers (Quarter Dog/ Melting Heart)	Recall a relationship that you are struggling with or a heartbreak that has been hard to get over. Bring compassion to where in your body you experience these sensations.

cont.

Organ pair (yin/ yang organs)	Physical	Emotional	Energetic	Mental	Yin pose (prototypes)	Yin inquiry
Spleen/Stomach	Extracts the essences of food and liquids and converts to blood and *Qi*. Filters blood, controls dampness, supports appetite, digestion, and absorption of nutrients	Grounded, calm, feeling at home in oneself, equanimity	Source of life for other organs, provides nourishment, controls cycles	Able to focus and concentrate, coherent thoughts and decisions	Front of legs (Saddle, Dragon) Twists (Dragonfly with a twist, Deer with twist)	Bring to mind a situation where you feel stuck, inflexible, or resistant. Notice how that feels in the body. Imagine taking an opposite action and notice how that feels in the body. Now, try to experience the sensations of both the resistance and opposite of this feeling (e.g., openness) at the same time in the body.
Lung/Large Intestine	Responsible for respiration, and flow of water including skin/ tissue processes and eliminates what is not needed	Perseverance, courage in the face of sadness, resolved grief	Tender organs that replenish energy, receives pure *Qi* and provides life through respiration	Tenacity, able to see the big picture, confidence, perseverance	Inner and outer arm (Quarter Dog/ Melting Heart) Chest (diaphragm/ lungs) (Fish, Snail)	If you are experiencing a recent loss or are having bouts of sadness, take a moment to recognize the sacredness of this experience. Notice where in your body you may need support, care, and tenderness, perhaps placing a hand on this area of the body and saying silently to yourself, "I am sorry, I love you."

DONNA'S STORY

Donna was a 26-year-old, white female, who had resided on an inpatient unit at my hospital for the past three years. She suffered from an eating disorder and Major Depression. I began working with Donna after a particularly low period for her. She had been on suicide watch for several weeks and was very sad, depressed, and discouraged. Donna and I started by practicing some very basic mindfulness meditation skills. She particularly resonated with loving-kindness and compassion practices, and I made a recording for her that she could use throughout the week.

Donna reported some relief from the practices and found that her thinking was more positive after a few weeks. She also enjoyed sharing the practices with her peers and started organizing a meditation group. We incorporated the inner resource so that she would have some tools when she began to struggle with negative feelings. She reported that her inner resource was the beach that she used to visit as a child where she felt happy and free. I asked her to practice this visualization daily to strengthen her connection to it whenever she needed it. Specifically, I encouraged her to use all of her senses in imagining herself at this beautiful beach.

In addition to her emotional difficulties, Donna struggled with obesity and was having trouble with her back, knees, and hips. I suggested that we might add some gentle yoga into our time together while still focusing on lovingkindness meditation. We started with chair yoga and did some gentle seated forward folds, hip openers, and twists. She was quite flexible and soon was able to take these same poses onto the floor. While in the poses, I asked her to create an intention for her body and mind in the present moment. She stated, "I am kind to my body." We practiced short lovingkindness meditations in each pose, taking time to strengthen positive emotions. Over time, her intention shifted to include compassion and lovingkindness for others. We slowly began to integrate energetic practices, including yin sequences that focused on different organ/meridian pairs. She particularly resonated with the Lung/Large Intestine sequence as this tapped into feelings of deep grief, sadness, and loss. Her tears, which had been so difficult for her to access while in the hospital, flowed freely when she was in a quiet pose. I often would just sit beside her with a gentle hand on her back as she cried and say, "I am sorry for your pain."

Her energy shifted after some of these sessions as she became more confident that she could be with her emotions and not fall apart. Instead of wanting to hurt herself, she began to treat her body with much more respect and care. She began losing weight and dressing with care, too. She continued to teach her peers different yin yoga practices as well, which seemed to strengthen her own inner resource. Donna eventually was discharged from the inpatient unit, and I continued to work with her in the step-down transitional program. She began attending yoga groups in the community and found a network of peers in a mental health advocacy group. When I asked Donna what supports helped her the most, she reflected that having a host of tools in her toolbox was most helpful because she could utilize some when she was struggling (inner resource) and others to strengthen her positive emotions (yin yoga, lovingkindness meditations).

ENDNOTES

1   iRest Resources (n.d.) www.irest.org/irest-research.

2   Hanson, R., and Mendius, R. (2009) *Buddha's Brain: The practical neuroscience of happiness, love and wisdom.* Oakland, CA: New Harbinger Publications.

3   Hanson, R. (2013) *Hardwiring Happiness: The new brain science of contentment, calm, and confidence.* New York: Harmony Books.

4   Hanson, R. (2013) *Hardwiring Happiness: The new brain science of contentment, calm, and confidence.* New York: Harmony Books, p.21.

5   Hanson, R. (2013) *Hardwiring Happiness: The new brain science of contentment, calm, and confidence.* New York: Harmony Books, p.21.

6   Hanson, R. (2013) *Hardwiring Happiness: The new brain science of contentment, calm, and confidence.* New York: Harmony Books.

7   Shatz, C.J. (1992) 'The developing brain.' *Scientific American, 267,* 60–67.

8   Seligman, M. (n.d.) Positive Psychology Center. https://ppc.sas.upenn.edu.

9   Fredrickson, B.L. (2001) 'The role of positive emotions in positive psychology. The broaden-and-build theory of positive emotions.' *American Psychologist, 56,* 3, 218–226.

10 Tugade, M.M., and Fredrickson, B.L. (2004) 'Resilient individuals use positive emotions to bounce back from negative emotional experiences.' *Journal of Personality and Social Psychology, 86,* 2, 320–333.

11 Zuo, X.L., Li, Q., Gao, F., Yang, L., and Meng, F.J. (2016) 'Effects of yoga on negative emotions in clients with breast cancer: A meta-analysis of randomized controlled trials.' *International Journal of Nursing Sciences, 3,* 299–306.

12 Ulger, O., and Yagli, N.V. (2010) 'Effect of yoga on quality of life in cancer clients.' *Complementary Therapies in Clinical Practice, 16,* 2, 60–63.

13 Kumar, N., Bhatnagar, S., Velpandian, T., Patnaik, S., *et al.* (2013) 'Randomized controlled trial in advance stage breast cancer clients for the effectiveness on stress marker and pain through sudarshan kriya and pranayama.' *Indian Journal of Palliative Care, 19,* 180–185.

14 Impett, E.A., Daubenmier, J.J., and Hirschman, A.L. (2006) 'Minding the body: Yoga, embodiment, and well-being.' *Sexual Research and Social Policy, 3,* 39–48.

15 Lavey, R., Sherman, T., Mueser, K.T., *et al.* (2005) 'The effects of yoga on mood in psychiatric inpatients.' *Psychiatric Rehabilitation Journal, 28,* 4, 399–402.

16 Ivtzan, I., and Papantoniou, A. (2014) 'Yoga meets positive psychology: Examining the integration of hedonic (gratitude) and eudaemonic (meaning) well-being in relation to the extent of yoga practice.' *Journal of Bodywork & Movement Therapies, 18,* 183–189.

17 Sullivan, M., Moonaz, S., Weber, K., Taylor, J., and Schmalzl, L. (2018) 'Toward an explanatory framework for yoga therapy informed by philosophical and ethical perspectives.' *Alternative Therapies in Health and Medicine, 24,* 1, 38–47.

18 Sullivan, M., Moonaz, S., Weber, K., Taylor, J., and Schmalzl, L. (2018) 'Toward an explanatory framework for yoga therapy informed by philosophical and ethical perspectives.' *Alternative Therapies in Health and Medicine, 24,* 1, 38–47.

19 Adele, D. (2009) *The Yamas and Niyamas: Exploring yoga's ethical practice.* Duluth, MN: On-Word Bound Books.

20 Stone, M. (2008) *The Inner Tradition of Yoga.* Boston, MA: Shambhala Publications.

21 Ram, B. (2009) *The Eight Limbs of Yoga: Pathway to liberation.* Coronado, CA: Deep Yoga.

22 Pantanjali (2003) *The Yoga-Sutra of Patanjali,* trans. Chip Hartranft. Boston, MA: Shambhala Publications, p.103.

23 Smith, J.A., Greer, T., Sheets, T., and Watson, S. (2011) 'Is there more to yoga than exercise?' *Alternative Therapies in Health and Medicine, 17,* 3, 22–29.

24 Kishida, M., Scherezade, M., Larkey, L., and Elavsky, S. (2018) 'Yoga resets my inner peace barometer: A qualitative study illuminating the pathways of how yoga impacts one's relationship to oneself and to others.' *Complementary Therapies in Medicine, 40,* 215–221.

25 Ross, A., Bevans, M., Friedmann, E., Williams, L., and Thomas, S.I. (2014) '"I am a nice person when I do yoga!!!": A qualitative analysis of how yoga affects relationships.' *Journal of Holistic Nursing, 32,* 2, 67–77.

26 Kinser, P.A., Bourguignon, C., Taylor, A.G., and Steeves, R. (2013) 'A feeling of connectedness: Perspectives on a gentle yoga intervention for women with major depression.' *Issues in Mental Health Nursing, 34,* 6, 402–411.

27 Dush, C.M.K., and Amator, P.R. (2005) 'Consequences of relationship status and quality for subjective well-being.' *Journal of Social and Personal Relationships, 22,* 607–627.

28 Kinser, P.A., Bourguignon, C., Taylor, A.G., and Steeves, R. (2013) 'A feeling of connectedness: Perspectives on a gentle yoga intervention for women with major depression.' *Issues in Mental Health Nursing, 34,* 6, 402–411.

29 iRest Resources (n.d.) www.irest.org/irest-research.

30 Shapiro, F. (2018) *Eye Movement Desensitization and Reprocessing (EMDR) Therapy: Basic principles, protocols, and procedures* (3rd ed.). New York: Guilford Press, p.117.

31 Kabat-Zinn, J. (1990) *Full Catastrophe Living: Using the wisdom of your body and mind to face stress, pain, and illness.* New York: Dell Publishing, p.XXXV.

32 Kabat-Zinn, J. (1990) *Full Catastrophe Living: Using the wisdom of your body and mind to face stress, pain, and illness.* New York: Dell Publishing, p.20.

33 Shapiro, S.L., and Carlson, L.E. (2009) *The Art and Science of Mindfulness: Integrating mindfulness into psychology and the helping professions.* Washington, DC: American Psychological Association, pp.8–9.

34 Shapiro, D.H. (1992) 'A preliminary study of long-term meditators: Goals, effects, religious orientation, cognitions.' *Journal of Transpersonal Psychology, 24,* 23–39.

35 Mackenzie, M.J., Carlson, L.E., Munoz, M., and Speca, M. (2007) 'A qualitative study of self-perceived effects of Mindfulness-based Stress Reduction (MBSR) in a psychosocial oncology setting.' *Stress and Health: Journal of the International Society for the Investigation of Stress, 23,* 1, 59–69.

36 Miller, R. (2015) *The iRest Program for Healing PTSD.* Oakland, CA: New Harbinger Publications, p.51.

37 Kaptchuk, T.J. (1983) *The Web That Has No Weaver: Understanding Chinese medicine.* New York: Congdon & Weed.

38 Beinfield, H., and Korngold, E. (1991) *Between Heaven and Earth: A guide to Chinese medicine.* New York: Random House.

39 Powers, S. (2008) *Insight Yoga.* Boulder, CO: Shambhala Publications.

40 Reichstein, G. (1998) *Wood Becomes Water: Chinese medicine in everyday life.* New York: Kodansha America.

41 Powers, S. (2008) *Insight Yoga.* Boulder, CO: Shambhala Publications.

42 Powers, S. (2008) *Insight Yoga.* Boulder, CO: Shambhala Publications.

43 Beinfield, H., and Korngold, E. (1991) *Between Heaven and Earth: A guide to Chinese medicine.* New York: Random House.

44 Kaptchuk, T.J. (1983) *The Web That Has No Weaver: Understanding Chinese medicine.* New York: Congdon & Weed.
45 Powers, S. (2008) *Insight Yoga.* Boulder, CO: Shambhala Publications.
46 Powers, S. (2008) *Insight Yoga.* Boulder, CO: Shambhala Publications.
47 https://joshsummers.net

— Chapter 6 —

BREATHING INTO YIN

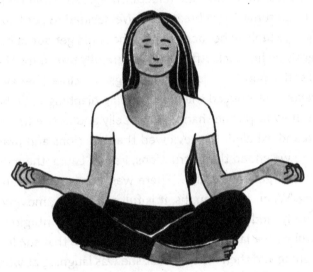

The optimal meditation position is one that allows both stability and ease

As a neuropsychologist, I have had the fortunate opportunity to be part of many of my clients' lives right from the beginning of their neurological injury (stroke, brain injury, brain tumor) recovery and then ongoing through the long slow process of rehabilitation and stabilization, which may extend for years. Laura is one client who I have been working with for the past 20 years. Laura has a severe brain injury and requires total care for all her activities of daily living, including bathing, dressing, toileting, and transfers. She is unable to eat and requires total nutrition through a feeding tube. She is not able to speak due to severe paralysis. She is able to write and spell out her thoughts, although it can be a time-consuming process. Over the years, I have utilized a variety of traditional cognitive behavioral approaches to help her adjust to her disability, anxiety, and family stressors. Recently, she began experiencing more anxiety as her physical health had started to decline. She was having more difficulty with her transfers getting in and out of her wheelchair, showering, and toileting. When I asked her to rate her anxiety on a scale of one to ten, she opened up both hands, indicating she was a ten out of ten.

I asked her if she was willing to try something different. She stared at me in a way that I knew well, and I said, "You are not sure you want to try something different, and you are tired of people trying to get you do things that you don't want to do." She nodded almost imperceptibly, and I knew that I was facing an uphill battle. Her sister, Laura's long-time caregiver and advocate, gently said, "Laura, why don't we try to do something different? We all need help with anxiety, and I will participate too." Her kind and warm tone seemed to soften Laura's resistance and she reluctantly agreed. I told them both that I would like to do some "yoga breathing." We decided to get Laura to her low physical therapy table in her bedroom so she could get out of her wheelchair and rest gently on her back. After we had carefully transferred her to the bed and placed soft supports underneath her legs, she closed her eyes and visibly began to relax. I introduced the idea of doing diaphragmatic breathing and showed her how to put her hand on her belly and notice its rise and fall as she inhaled and exhaled. We reviewed the directions and practiced a few times. Before we ended the instructions, I said, "Laura, the most important thing is don't forget to breathe." There was a pause and then Laura burst out laughing. When Laura laughs, it is full and robust, moving throughout her entire body, and lasts for several minutes. It is contagious and makes everyone around her laugh as well, since it is so rare that she lets herself go. I began laughing and then realized that she was laughing at what I had said! She was thinking, "Of course I will not forget to breathe. No one forgets to breathe or they are dead!" We laughed together for a few more moments and then she settled and relaxed on her table. I began breathing with her, gently reminding her, her mom, and myself not to forget to notice our breath and appreciate every breath that allows us to remain alive even amidst so much struggle and suffering. Each breath reminds us of our aliveness.

In yin yoga, the role of the breath has many possible applications. Observation of the breath (mindfulness), breath enhancement (pranayama), and breath for relaxation can all be utilized in a yin practice to support the practitioner in their specific intentions, goals, and outcomes for the practice. For example, a yoga practitioner may want to enhance their ability to stay in the present moment during the yoga class, so they may benefit from mindfulness of the breath practice. Another yogi may feel tired and dull, and benefit from applying kapalabhati (breath enhancing with belly pumping) to refresh their energy during a yin pose. To return to the metaphor that yin is like tofu, breath practices are like spices that help to "season" the tofu to enhance the benefit to the practitioner—whether they want more energy, more mental stability, or better relaxation.

Mindfulness of breathing has been taught for thousands of years, beginning with some of the earliest Buddhist teachings. As a form of meditation, mindfulness of breathing (called *anapanasati* in the ancient texts) was a way to establish concentration and was considered one of the most important steps toward enlightenment.[1] The author Analayo, who translated the ancient text *Satipatthana*, describes how "The Buddha himself frequently engaged in mindfulness of breathing, which he called a 'noble' and 'divine' way of practicing."[2] The practice of *anapanasati* has been detailed at great length in the ancient texts and can be simplified by understanding this method as *one-pointed focused attention* on the *in-breath and out-breath*.

My teacher, Sarah Powers, describes how this practice of mindfulness of the breath "brings us into a direct relationship with the roots of suffering (our patterns of reactivity) and ultimately stimulates insight into our deeper wisdom nature."[3] There are many helpful texts that readers may find useful if they are interested in learning more about the philosophical underpinnings of mindfulness. These include Analayo, *Satipatthana*;[4] Bhikkhu Bodhi, *In the Buddha's Words*;[5] Huston Smith and Philip Novak, *Buddhism: A concise introduction*;[6] Rupert Gethin, *The Foundations of Buddhism*;[7] Bhante Guanaratana, *Mindfulness in Plain English*;[8] and Sarah Powers, *Insight Yoga*.[9]

Mindfulness training usually begins with the breath as it is the easiest and most accessible way to examine our experience directly. The Buddhist teachings describe four foundations or "interrelated domains of experience" that can further support the alleviation of suffering and lead to ultimate enlightenment.[10] The four foundations (also known as four contemplations) are described in the ancient text *Satipatthana* as the following:

1. Contemplation of the body, including mindfulness of the breath and the body postures
2. Contemplation of feeling, including three primary types: pleasant, unpleasant, and neutral
3. Contemplation of the mind, including mental states or moods
4. Contemplation of phenomena or mind objects, including the mind sensations or the way that the mind observes changing phenomena.[11, 12]

Religious scholars Huston Smith and Philip Novak describe how these four foundations of mindfulness not only help with calming the mind and increasing concentration, but also act "as a platform for vipassana, a special kind of self-observation or inner empiricism that produces 'penetrative seeing.'"[13] This is often described as *insight*. The potent combination of concentration and insight can lead to what Smith and Novak describe as "the path to freedom."[14] Each of these foundations can be an important exploration for yin yoga students as they discover more "insights" about their experience with their body in different physical postures (first foundation); detect the feelings associated with the sensations (second foundation); observe the flow of emotions in yin shapes (third foundation); and notice the changing sensations from pose to pose along with their changing thoughts/feelings/emotions (fourth foundation).

In modern teachings, paying attention to the breath is considered a simple yet powerful way to cultivate moment-to-moment awareness in the present moment. There are different places in the body one can focus on when paying attention to the breath. These include the nostrils from which the air is moving in and out, the chest as the lungs expand and relax, and the belly that can move in and out with each breath. Jon Kabat-Zinn describes how in Mindfulness-Based Stress Reduction (MBSR) "we generally focus on the sensations of breathing at the belly rather than at the nostrils or in the chest. This is partly because doing so tends to be particularly relaxing and calming in the early stages of practice."[15] In addition, when we focus on the breath, it is a reliable and readily available anchor. We don't have to search out or strain to find the breath. According to researchers, the average person takes between 17,280 and 23,040 breaths a day.[16] However, we often don't pay attention to even one full breath. By turning toward the breath, we can quiet the mind. Kabat-Zinn says, "resting in awareness of the breath sensations, even for a moment or two, we are out of the wind and protected from the buffeting action of the waves and their tension-producing effects. This is an extremely effective way to reconnect with the potential for calmness within you."[17]

In yin yoga, mindfulness of the breath can be a vital tool to help students stay connected to the present moment. In holding poses for long periods, the mind can easily wander. I have had that experience myself many times of going into a pose and after a minute, finding that my mind has started going into planning mode, thinking about my grocery list, bills, or whatever is the recurrent worry for the day. That is a signal to me that I need to strengthen my concentration, and I return to the simple and effective practice of awareness of breath. This is important for students to get the full benefit from a yin pose. Even if their bodies are receiving the tugging and pulling on the connective tissue, if yoga students are not present in the here and now, they will miss some of the most important aspects of the yin pose, namely present-moment feedback from the pose.

How can students know if the sensations are too strong or not strong enough if their minds are on something else? Mindfulness of the breath can support a much safer and stabilizing practice as students adjust the level of sensation while becoming much more aware of the entire body once their attention is more "gathered." Mindfulness of the breath during a yin pose can also help enhance the positive physical benefits of the pose. The body stays in a more receptive state so that it is easier to stay still long enough for the potent tugging and loading on the connective tissues to occur. In addition, once concentration is strengthened with regular practice, students can explore more subtle practices, including the four foundations of mindfulness.

The connection between breath and yoga can be traced back to the earliest writings on yoga nearly 2000 years ago. In Patanjali's *Yoga Sutras,* or scriptures, one of the earliest ancient spiritual texts written about yoga sometime between 500 BCE and 400 CE, the sage Pantajali describes how breath can be a powerful practice toward stilling the body and mind.[18, 19, 20]

"*Pranayama* (literally 'breath energy' plus 'discipline, restraint') is generally regarded today as a set of practices in which one consciously directs the breath and its energies in deliberate patterns."[21] *Pranayama* can be characterized both by simple practices as described in the Sutras, and by very complex patterns of breathing that evolved in later schools of yoga, including tantric and Tibetan practices. Over the centuries, yogis have recognized the benefits of practicing *pranayama* as a form of healthy living. By focusing on a combination of timed sequences for inhalation, exhalation, and suspension of breath, we "not only strengthen our prana, we vitalize the body right down to the cellular level."[22]

Yoga scholar Bhava Ram describes how the science behind *pranayama* is related to the autonomic nervous system, or the balance between the sympathetic and parasympathetic nervous systems. Regular *pranayama* practice can facilitate relaxation. He says, "when relaxed, the mind produces alpha waves which are more flowing, smooth and even. All true healing is based upon this relaxation, as are all true spiritual practices. *Pranayama* facilitates our entering into the alpha state."[23] Stephen Cope, renowned psychotherapist and yoga teacher, in his beautiful depiction of the healing power of yoga in *Yoga and the Quest for the True Self,* writes, "Yogis describes the breath as lying precisely at the boundary between the body and the mind. Breath is seen as the bridge to the energy body and to the emotion body, which is an aspect of it."[24] For more background on the history of *pranayama,* I recommend Ram's text *The Eight Limbs of Yoga,*[25] Chip Hartranft's translation of *The Yoga-Sutra of Patanjali,*[26] the late yoga teacher Michael Stone's *The Inner Tradition of Yoga,*[27] and Stephen Cope's book *Yoga and the Quest of the True Self.*[28] For research on *pranayama* and mental health, many different types of *pranayama* practice have been explored that have demonstrated a positive benefit of various breath practices on physical and mental health.[29, 30, 31] Some of these studies need to be replicated in larger groups, but the early work is quite promising in terms of the power of breath to support well-being. Please also see Dr. Richard Brown and Dr. Patricia Gerbarg's work on yogic breathing in psychiatric care for further reading on this topic.[32, 33, 34, 35]

Pranayama practices continue to be an integral part of 21st-century yoga. Most yoga classes, yoga teacher training programs, and yoga therapy sessions contain some form of *pranayama* practice. The following list is not exhaustive but contains many of the commonly utilized *pranayama* practices that can be sequenced in a yin yoga session. Some of the practices are better known by their Sanskrit names (this is the ancient language used in early yoga texts), which are italicized. These practices include deep diaphragmatic breathing; yogic three-part breath or *dirgha* (taking a slow and full inhale as though you are breathing into the belly, lower chest, and upper chest); equalized breath or *sama vritti* (matching the length of the inhale and exhale), victorious breath or *ujjayi* (breathing in and out of the nose with gentle constriction of the back of the throat, creating an ocean-like sound); alternate nostril breathing or *nadishodona* (closing off one nostril; inhaling and exhaling through the open nostril; repeating on the opposite side); forceful breathing or *kapalabhati* (alternating long passive inhalations followed by short, forceful out-breaths by contracting the lower belly and pushing out air from the lungs); Bellows Breath or *bhastrika* (rapidly inhaled air that is forcefully exhaled while contracting the lower belly and pushing out air from the lungs); vibrational breathing or *bhramari* breath (an audible humming sound is made on the exhale while keeping the lips and ears closed by placing index fingers on ears right at the cartilage).

What makes the use of *pranayama* different in yin classes than in traditional flow or yang yoga classes is the *purpose* and *intention* for the breath work. In flow classes, *pranayama* can be used for a variety of purposes, including to increase energy levels, to get through difficult poses, to relax and release tension—these are just a few of the many benefits. In yin, *pranayama* is used to maximize the *therapeutic benefit* of the pose. For example, equalized breath can help gather attention and ease anxiety while in a backbend pose such as Sphinx, so that the participant is able to stay focused for the entire duration of the pose. Rather than trying to change the sensations of the pose or increase the intensity, in yin we are simply using the breath to help support us in staying connected to what is happening in the current moment. Even more intense *pranayama* practices such as *kapalabhati* can be used as a support in a yin pose, particularly for more challenging shapes such as Frog pose. By gently contracting the belly during the exhalation and finding a stabilizing rhythm of the breath, Frog pose can become more accessible as the mind finds a focal point to stay connected to the breath and sensations in the body. Even if the *pranayama* practice does not result in an expected response, the student has important material to explore as part of an inquiry practice.

THE ART AND SCIENCE OF BREATH

While the ancient yogis and Buddhist meditators have been utilizing the breath to create a sense of well-being for more than two centuries, Western science only began to explore the healing potential of the breath in the later part of the 20th century. In 1974, Herbert Benson, a physician and pioneer in mind-body medicine at Harvard, described the *relaxation response*,[36] which included both physiological and emotional responses occurring as a result of a specific form of meditation (transcendental meditation that uses breath awareness along with mantra). He reported that practicing this form of meditation can promote better health, including reduced blood pressure and resting heart rate, and can lead to a sense of well-being.[37, 38, 39] His ability to demonstrate with scientific rigor that meditation has a profound influence on the mind and body set the stage for the growing field of integrative and complementary medicine in the 21st century. Researchers have continued to explore how different types of breathing can impact how we think (cognition), feel (emotions), and act (behavior). In particular, there is a substantial body of research supporting the power of coherent breathing.[40, 41, 42, 43, 44, 45] According to Dr. Richard Brown and Dr. Patricia Gerbarg, "coherent breathing is a simple way to increase heart-rate variability and balance the stress-response system."[46]

What Brown and Gerbarg and others have discovered is the important connection between the pattern of the heart rate and the nervous system. When the heart rate is smoother and more regular through the practice of slow breathing exercises, more positive emotions are typically experienced.[47, 48] By slowing the breath down to an average of about five breaths per minute, the heart rate variability (HRV) increases. Higher HRV is associated with a more balanced stress-response system, healthier cardiovascular functioning, and greater health.[49] There are many different programs that promote coherent breathing, including HeartMath,[50] Breath-Body-Mind,[51] and Coherent Breathing for Health.[52]

Coherent breathing is often utilized during yoga practices and can have benefits for mental health wellness and depression.[53, 54, 55] In yin yoga, coherent breathing can be helpful to support nervous system balance, especially when there is "healthy" stress during a pose that might activate the sympathetic nervous system and create tension in the body that makes it harder for the yoga student to relax and open into the sensations. By using coherent breathing in a long-held pose (Saddle pose, for example), students can regulate their responses by slowing the breath down to maintain good heart rate variability and avoid a sudden trigger into a stress response. As students relax and hold the pose, the breath may even lengthen more (from a count of five breaths per minute to two or three), creating a feeling of ease that can remain after they come out of the pose.

In my experience, yin yoga provides the canvas to explore different breath "art forms," including mindfulness, *pranayama*, and coherent breathing. For beginners, I start with mindfulness of the breath, as it is most accessible and helps my clients to strengthen their present-moment awareness to maximize the benefit of the yin practice. As they become more comfortable with gathering attention and tracking sensations in the body, I introduce more subtle energetic *pranayama* practices. It is important not to have a specific agenda with *pranayama* (e.g., if my clients do *kapalabhati*, they will feel more energized), but rather allowing them to be curious and explore how the breath practice is landing inside of them. The use of inquiry is helpful, especially when introducing a new practice to clients. Here are some simple questions to stimulate the inquiry process:

- How is my breath practice affecting me moment to moment?
- How did the breath practice impact me at the end of my yoga practice?
- What was the impact of the breath practice on the rest of my day?
- Are there any breath practices that I would like to continue off the yoga mat?

ENDNOTES

1   Bodhi, B. (2005) *In the Buddha's Words: An anthology of discourses from the Pāli canon.* Boston, MA: Wisdom Publications.
2   Analayo (2008) *Satipatthana.* Cambridge: Windhorse Publications, p.125.
3   Powers, S. (2008) *Insight Yoga.* Boulder, CO: Shambhala Publications, pp.174.
4   Analayo (2008) *Satipatthana.* Cambridge: Windhorse Publications.
5   Bodhi, B. (2005) *In the Buddha's Words: An anthology of discourses from the Pāli canon.* Boston, MA: Wisdom Publications.
6   Smith, H., and Novak, P. (2003) *Buddhism: A concise introduction.* New York: HarperCollins Publishers.

7   Gethin, R. (1998) *The Foundations of Buddhism.* Oxford: Oxford University Press.
8   Gunaratana, H. (2019) *Mindfulness in Plain English.* Somerville, MA: Wisdom Publications.
9   Powers, S. (2008) *Insight Yoga.* Boulder, CO: Shambhala Publications.
10 Powers, S. (2008) *Insight Yoga.* Boulder, CO: Shambhala Publications.
11 Bodhi, B. (2005) *In the Buddha's Words: An anthology of discourses from the Pāli canon.* Boston, MA: Wisdom Publications.
12 Gunaratana, H. (2019) *Mindfulness in Plain English.* Somerville, MA: Wisdom Publications.
13 Smith, H., and Novak, P. (2003) *Buddhism: A concise introduction.* New York: HarperCollins Publishers, p.79.
14 Smith, H., and Novak, P. (2003) *Buddhism: A concise introduction.* New York: HarperCollins Publishers, p.79.
15 Zinn-Kabat, J. (2013) *Full Catastrophe Living: Using the wisdom of your body and mind to face stress, pain, and illness.* New York: Bantam Publishers, p.45.
16 Brown, A. (2014) 'How many breaths do you take each day?' https://blog.epa.gov/2014/04/28/how-many-breaths-do-you-take-each-day.
17 Zinn-Kabat, J. (2013) *Full Catastrophe Living: Using the wisdom of your body and mind to face stress, pain, and illness.* New York: Bantam Publishers, p.45.
18 Cope, S. (1999) *Yoga and the Quest for the True Self.* New York: Bantam Publications.
19 Hartranft, C. (2003) *The Yoga-Sutra of Pantanjali.* Boston, MA: Shambhala Publications.
20 Ram, B. (2009) *The Eight Limbs of Yoga.* Twin Lakes, WI: Lotus Press.
21 Hartranft, C. (2003) *The Yoga-Sutra of Pantanjali.* Boston, MA: Shambhala Publications, p.40.
22 Hartranft, C. (2003) *The Yoga-Sutra of Pantanjali.* Boston, MA: Shambhala Publications, p.40.
23 Ram, B. (2009) *The Eight Limbs of Yoga.* Twin Lakes, WI: Lotus Press, p.152.
24 Cope, S. (1999) *Yoga and the Quest for the True Self.* New York: Bantam Publications, p.206.
25 Ram, B. (2009) *The Eight Limbs of Yoga.* Twin Lakes, WI: Lotus Press.
26 Hartranft, C. (2003) *The Yoga-Sutra of Pantanjali.* Boston, MA: Shambhala Publications.
27 Stone, M. (2008) *The Inner Tradition of Yoga.* Boston, MA: Shambhala Publications.
28 Cope, S. (1999) *Yoga and the Quest for the True Self.* New York: Bantam Publications.
29 Kuppusamy, K., Kamaldeen, D., Pitani, R., Amaldas, J., and Shanmugam, P. (2018) 'Effects of Bhramari Pranayama on health: A systematic review.' *Journal of Traditional and Complementary Medicine, 8,* 11–16.
30 Franklin, R., Butler, M., and Bentley, J. (2018) 'The physical postures of yoga practices may protect against depressive symptoms, even as life stressors increase: A moderation analysis.' *Psychology, Health, & Medicine, 23,* 7, 870–890.
31 Streeter, C.C., Gerbarg, P.L., Whitfield, T.H., *et al.* (2017) 'Treatment of major depressive disorder with iyengar yoga and coherent breathing: A randomized controlled dosing study.' *Alternative & Complementary Therapies: A New Bimonthly Publication for Health Care Practitioners, 23,* 6, 236–243.
32 Brown, R.P., and Gerbarg, P.L. (2016) 'Neurobiology and neurophysiology of breath practices in psychiatric care.' *Psychiatric Times, 33,* 11, 22–25.
33 Brown, R.P., and Gerbarg, P.L. (2005) 'Sudarshan Kriya yogic breathing in the treatment of stress, anxiety, and depression. Part I – Neurophysiologic model.' *Journal of Alternative and Complementary Medicine, 11,* 1, 189–201.
34 Brown, R.P., and Gerbarg, P.L. (2005) 'Sudarshan Kriya Yogic breathing in the treatment of stress, anxiety, and depression. Part II – Clinical applications and guidelines.' *Journal of Alternative and Complementary Medicine, 11,* 4, 711–717.
35 Scott, T.M., Gerbarg, P.L., Silveri, M.M., *et al.* (2019) 'Psychological function, iyengar yoga, and coherent breathing: A randomized controlled dosing study.' *Journal of Psychiatric Practice, 25,* 6, 437–450.
36 Benson, H., and Klipper, M.Z. (1975) *The Relaxation Response.* New York: Avon.
37 Benson, H., Beary, J.F., and Carol, M.P. (1975) 'The relaxation response.' *Psychiatry, 37,* 1, 37–45.

38 Wallace, R.K., Benson, H., and Wilson, A.F. (1971) 'A wakeful hypometabolic physiological state.' *American Journal of Physiology, 221,* 3, 795–799.

39 Benson, H. (1997) 'The relaxation response: Therapeutic effects.' *Science, 278,* 5344, 1694–1695.

40 Franklin, R., Butler, M., and Bentley, J. (2018) 'The physical postures of yoga practices may protect against depressive symptoms, even as life stressors increase: A moderation analysis.' *Psychology, Health, & Medicine, 23,* 7, 870–890.

41 Streeter, C.C., Gerbarg, P.L., Whitfield, T.H., *et al.* (2017) 'Treatment of major depressive disorder with iyengar yoga and coherent breathing: A randomized controlled dosing study.' *Alternative & Complementary Therapies: A New Bimonthly Publication for Health Care Practitioners, 23,* 6, 236–243.

42 Scott, T.M., Gerbarg, P.L., Silveri, M.M., *et al.* (2019) 'Psychological function, iyengar yoga, and coherent breathing: A randomized controlled dosing study.' *Journal of Psychiatric Practice, 25,* 6, 437–450.

43 Benson, H. (1997) 'The relaxation response: Therapeutic effects.' *Science, 278,* 5344, 1694–1695.

44 Brown, R., and Gerbarg, P. (2012) *The Healing Power of the Breath.* Boulder, CO: Shambhala Publications.

45 Brown, R.P., Gerbarg, P.L., and Meunch, F. (2013) 'Breathing practices for treatment of psychiatric and stress-related medical conditions.' *Psychiatric Clinics of North America, 36,* 121–140.

46 Brown, R., and Gerbarg, P. (2012) *The Healing Power of the Breath.* Boulder, CO: Shambhala Publications, p.12.

47 Brown, R., and Gerbarg, P. (2012) *The Healing Power of the Breath.* Boulder, CO: Shambhala Publications.

48 Brown, R.P., Gerbarg, P.L., and Meunch, F. (2013) 'Breathing practices for treatment of psychiatric and stress-related medical conditions.' *Psychiatric Clinics of North America, 36,* 121–140.

49 Brown, R.P., Gerbarg, P.L., and Meunch, F. (2013) 'Breathing practices for treatment of psychiatric and stress-related medical conditions.' *Psychiatric Clinics of North America, 36,* 121–140.

50 www.heartmath.com/hm-2

51 www.breath-body-mind.com

52 https://coherentbreathing.com

53 Franklin, R., Butler, M., and Bentley, J. (2018) 'The physical postures of yoga practices may protect against depressive symptoms, even as life stressors increase: A moderation analysis.' *Psychology, Health, & Medicine, 23,* 7, 870–890.

54 Streeter, C.C., Gerbarg, P.L., Whitfield, T.H., *et al.* (2017) 'Treatment of major depressive disorder with iyengar yoga and coherent breathing: A randomized controlled dosing study.' *Alternative & Complementary Therapies: A New Bimonthly Publication for Health Care Practitioners, 23,* 6, 236–243.

55 Scott, T.M., Gerbarg, P.L., Silveri, M.M., *et al.* (2019) 'Psychological function, iyengar yoga, and coherent breathing: A randomized controlled dosing study.' *Journal of Psychiatric Practice, 25,* 6, 437–450.

Chapter 7

EASING SUFFERING THROUGH YIN YOGA

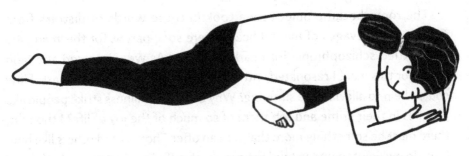

Sleeping Swan invites a graceful surrender in the sensations of the hips

As a clinical psychologist in a psychiatric hospital, I was often called in to work with clients who had "behavioral issues." These issues could be extreme, ranging from physical and verbal aggression to suicidal ideation and self-harm (e.g., cutting, ingesting and inserting foreign bodies into various orifices of the body). I met Thomas for the first time at a treatment team meeting. These meetings are held monthly at the hospital and include the nursing staff, psychiatrist, psychologist, social worker, rehabilitation staff, advocates, the client, and their family. The team usually meets for a few minutes before the client arrives to review care, issues of concern, and treatment goals. That day, the team began to review Thomas's progress over the last month, and each provider agreed that he was not doing well. He was becoming increasingly paranoid around staff, refusing to take his medications because he thought he was being poisoned, and no longer participating in any therapy groups. What was even more concerning was that he had punched a peer on the unit the previous day because the man came into the bathroom and "got too close to me." His psychiatrist was considering an increase in his medications and wanted me to start working with Thomas on a behavioral plan to increase compliance.

As soon as Thomas came into the small conference room, I knew I was in for a challenge. He was a tall man in his mid-50s with graying blond hair. He was disheveled, dressed in sweatpants and a stained sweatshirt. He had a strong body odor, and it was clear that he had not changed his clothing or bathed in a while. He sat at the table with his treatment team, and the doctor reviewed his concerns and raised the idea of increasing his medications. Thomas slammed his hands down on the table, causing everyone to jump. "You are trying to kill me!" he shouted. The doctor calmly reassured him that the team was here to help him and told him to please relax and calm down. Thomas responded to the doctor's calm voice and reassuring demeanor by putting his head in his hands and starting to cry quietly. After a few minutes, he looked up at the team and shook his head sadly.

"I am suffering."

The room became quiet as we took in these words of distress from Thomas. The ravages of mental health were so apparent for this man who had battled schizophrenia for nearly 40 years. As we witnessed and held space for this man, I resonated with his deep despair and helplessness. How could I help to alleviate his suffering? Why did mental illness strike people like Thomas in their prime and rob them of so much of the joy of life? I thought, there must be something more that we can offer Thomas and others like him. It made me want to understand the nature of suffering. As a new mindfulness student, I was immediately drawn to the Buddhist teachings around suffering, beginning with the Four Noble Truths.

The Four Noble Truths are the foundation of Buddhist teachings. The Buddha's first formal discourse was said to be on this topic after his six-year-long search for enlightenment. The Four Noble Truths are often described as an answer to life's most important questions that spiritual seekers will ask when they begin their path. The First Noble Truth starts with the tenet that life is *dukkha*, translated from the Pali language of the Buddhist teachings to mean suffering.[1] For many people, this seems like an extremely pessimistic view of life that not only provides little comfort about our human existence but can actually lead to feelings of despair and hopelessness. However, a more nuanced look at this idea of *dukkha* can provide a deeper and perhaps more meaningful perspective. *Dukkha* is sometimes translated as "dissatisfaction," "tension," or a sense of "discontent." Interestingly, this definition suggests that *dukkha* can simply come from the recognition that something we love is coming to an end. Gregory Kramer, one of my Buddhist teachers, describes how we make a mistake when we don't want to look at suffering head on because of the fear that we may get overwhelmed or frightened. He says that in reality the opposite is true: "Looking clearly at the fact of suffering is one of the small number of things we can actually do that, together, bring real relief."[2] The clarity that comes from observing life directly and realistically can lead us to a path of discovery, connection, and openheartedness. Gregory Kramer aptly describes this process: "To observe life this directly is not pessimistic, it is realistic. Ignoring the problem doesn't help. Indeed, ignorance keeps the suffering invisible, assures its continuity, and establishes it as determining the tenor of our lives."[3] When I learned about the Four Noble Truths, instead of feeling hopeless, I actually felt relieved. I knew I was not alone in my suffering, fears, and anxieties. I felt more connected to my fellow humans who are struggling just as I am. I recognized that I am no different than my client Thomas, my friends, and my family. We are all in this life together, struggling, suffering, and wanting to find ease.

I have heard the Buddha described as a philosopher and spiritual leader, as well as the first clinical psychologist. He explored the challenges of being human and the psychological and physical suffering that is naturally part of being born, growing old, and dying. Like any good psychologist, he understood the importance of a solid clinical diagnosis, how the diagnosis came to be, and most importantly, how to construct and implement a good treatment plan to reduce suffering. The Four Noble Truths lay out this *diagnostic and treatment workup.*

The Second Noble Truth helps us to understand *why we suffer* or what causes suffering that leads us to a complicated and sometimes painful existence. The cause of life's suffering is what the Buddha describes as *tanha,* which can be translated as desire or hunger.[4] Such desires or hungers cause us to seek sensory pleasures like sex, food, or longing for love, that create an impulse of grasping for more as soon as one experiences them. On the other side, aversion or movement away from physical and emotional or psychological pain can also create suffering—like with my client, Thomas, who was constantly trying to get his psychotic symptoms to go away. According to the Buddha, this tension between grasping and aversion is the source of human suffering, whether it is addiction, physical or mental illness, or heartbreak when a relationship ends.

The Third Noble Truth becomes the therapeutic treatment plan of the Buddha's teachings. After laying out the truth of suffering and its causes, he logically arrives at how to find relief from suffering, which is both simple and profound: it is the cessation of this cycle of craving and aversion that naturally leads to the end of suffering. This sounds deceptively easy. How are we supposed to stop our desires and hungers? Of course, the Buddha anticipated this challenge, as it is a natural part of our human conditioning to fail to see beyond our own personal narrative, to feel separate and alone in our struggles and suffering. To work with the challenges of this separate self and the narrow lens that obscures the possibilities of living a happier life, the Buddha says that cessation of suffering does not happen all at once, but instead fades and lessens over time. As the tension abates, even just a little, we start to feel better. However, we need tools to help us release the grip of our desires. Just identifying them and wanting to feel better is not enough. Gregory Kramer says,

> The Buddha recognized that specific actions and conditions were needed to turn the possibility of freedom into an actuality, and he described them clearly in his fundamental teaching he called the Noble Eightfold Path, a path common to all schools of Buddhism that is also attractive to non-Buddhists. His "noble" path addresses the whole of our lives, from everyday actions to the most refined meditative practices.[5]

The Path is made up of "eight significant dimensions of one's behavior—mental, spoken, and bodily—that are regarded as operating dependently with one another and defining a complete way of living."[6] These dimensions include: *right view, right intention, right speech, right action, right livelihood, right effort, right mindfulness*, and *right concentration.* The term *right* refers not to a moral weight or judgment, but instead to the collective transformation that occurs as the eight dimensions are established and practiced over time, moving us away from suffering and toward freedom. In contrast, *wrong* view suggests engaging in behaviors that lead away from well-being, wholeness, and enlightenment.

There are many wonderful resources that describe the Noble Eightfold Path in accessible language that can be applied to everyday life. Two of my favorites are Bhante Gunaratana's book *Eight Mindful Steps to Happiness,*[7] and Gregory Kramer's book *A Whole-Life Path.*[8]

To make the Eightfold Path come to life, I like to do practices that awaken curiosity and reflection in different aspects of the path. Yin yoga can provide a framework to begin to explore different dimensions. I will sometimes stay with one dimension throughout a practice or a series of practices. For example, I will teach on the Four Noble Truths over a period of four weeks, with an exploration of each "truth" as the theme for that week. Table 7.1 shows different practices that can be done in the context of a yin class. The chart includes both philosophical and psychological descriptions of the dimensions of behavior. The philosophical descriptions include the traditional Buddhist meaning of each dimension along with the three cardinal points (which are the most essential principles distilled down from the eight dimensions, including wisdom, conduct, and meditation). The yin poses can be modified to enhance the inquiry practice for each individual.

Table 7.1 Eightfold Path and yin yoga

Eight dimensions of behaviors	Traditional meaning	Three cardinal points	Psychological meaning	Practices in yin yoga
Right view	Recognizing the Four Noble Truths	Wisdom (*prajna*)	Understanding what can increase suffering and what can reduce suffering on both a personal and a global level	While in a yin shape, explore the following contemplations: What is arising as I take this shape and stay for a while? Notice thoughts that pull you away or toward another thought (grasping vs. aversion). Notice sensations in the body that pull you away or toward action (grasping vs. aversion).
Right intention	With right view, we create intentions and aspirations from the heart that are wholesome	Wisdom	We consciously reinforce responses that align with and support our larger intentions (e.g., compassion, friendliness) and release those that don't (e.g., anger, jealousy)	While in a yin shape, explore the following contemplations: Select a yin pose that provides a sense of ease and support (e.g., Reclining Butterfly). Resolve to practice unconditional kindness toward yourself by finding ease in the body, breath, and mind. When the mind wanders or moves toward aversion, gently return to kindness. Notice if aversion remains, bring loving attention to the aversion, and acknowledge the discomfort that remains.
Right speech	Communication that includes speech that is timely, kind, helpful, and wise along with skillful listening	Conduct (*Sila*)	Speech can have a powerful effect for both the speaker and receiver. If done mindfully, it leads to skillful, friendly, and wholesome interpersonal communication	While in a yin shape, explore the following contemplations: Choose a yin pose that you do not typically select that might not give you as much ease (e.g., Frog pose). As you take the shape, begin to mentally note the different thoughts and feelings that arise. Notice how this inner speech affects you. Consider whether the words you say to yourself are harmful to you, or helpful, or neutral. Would these same words spoken to someone else harm or help or bring benefit to them?

cont.

Eight dimensions of behaviors	Three cardinal points	Traditional meaning	Psychological meaning	Practices in yin yoga
Right action	Conduct	Actions or non-harming (refraining from killing, stealing, or sexual misconduct) that lead to the welfare of ourselves and others	Reduce behaviors that can harm self or others and engage in wholesome behaviors that create inner stability	While in a yin shape, explore the following contemplations: Choose a yin shape that allows you to explore the "edge" of sensation safely (e.g., Butterfly pose). After taking the shape, find your edge and notice the impact on the body/mind/heart as you stay for at least 5–10 breaths. Slowly work toward the outermost range of the edge, while still keeping the body safe. Notice the impact on the body/mind/heart as you stay for at least 5–10 breaths. Notice how this action may have shifted the physical and emotional feedback you are receiving. Finally, return back to the edge that feels most beneficial and once again reflect on how this action impacts your physical and emotional state.
Right livelihood	Conduct	Work that supports a wholesome path and societal harmony, avoiding types of business that engage in harmful practices, or that promote killing or societal destruction	Create a livelihood that contributes to the greater good on an individual and collective level, or support and enable others to engage in wholesome actions to create a better society	While in a yin shape, explore the following contemplations: Come into a side-lying position over a bolster, extending the arms overhead and hands together in prayer position. Sense in the body the nourishing qualities of the pose. How does this pose foster a sense of comfort or safety? Notice if you need to adjust your position or add a prop (block under the hands to raise the floor). Reflect on how a sense of comfort and ease plays out in daily life. Does it create more harmony in your personal and work life? Consider times when you have felt ill at ease. How does that impact your personal and work life? Reflect on what you say "yes" to and "no" to in your personal and work life. Does it promote a sense of ease and well-being or tightness and constriction?

Right effort	Actions that prevent or abandon unwholesome states and initiate and maintain wholesome states	Meditation	To direct effort in a sustainable balanced way to create positive change and strengthen one's purpose and mission	While in a yin shape, explore the following contemplations: Take Seal pose (if available and safe for shoulders; Sphinx can be an alternative). Notice the sensations in the body in this pose. Consider the amount of "effort" it requires to stay in the shape. Is it sustainable? If is not, what modifications are needed to create balance and maintain the shape? Once you have found balance, notice what happens to your thoughts and emotions. Is there a sense of balance or separateness?
Right mindfulness	Meditations on the Four Foundations; body, feelings, mind, and mental objects (e.g., Four Noble Truths, mental hindrances)	Meditation	Reducing everyday suffering through mindfulness practice, which serves to cultivate compassion, kindness, and clarity	While in a yin shape, explore the following contemplations: Come into Butterfly or Butterfly with Legs Up the Wall. Notice the sensations of the breath and body. Take a few moments and observe how the sensations come and go. Next, shift your awareness to your feelings. Take a few moments and observe the different feeling tones. Next, shift to observe your thoughts, observing the coming and going of thoughts without getting stuck on one particular thought. Finally, observe any hindrances or barriers that are interfering with mindful awareness. Name that hindrance (e.g., worried thought) and perhaps acknowledge that there is suffering present. Finally, allow open awareness for thoughts, feelings, and body sensations to come and go.
Right concentration	The mind is gathered, and concentration is refined	Meditation	Greater and greater stillness of the mind leads to a deep sense of calmness, contentment, and gratitude	While in a yin shape, explore the following contemplations: Come into Relaxation pose (Savasana or Legs Up the Wall). Allow the body to come into stillness. Using the breath as anchor, begin to find stability of the mind. Now, consider all the things you are grateful for today. Reflect on small and large aspects (from the food you ate for breakfast to a loving connection with a dear friend) As you reflect on these, notice what happens to the mind. Notice a sense of contentment and how that affects the body. If the mind wanders, just gently direct the attention back to this sense of contentment and ease.

ENDNOTES

1   Smith, H., and Novak, P. (2003) *Buddhism: A concise introduction.* New York: Harper San Francisco.

2   Kramer, G. (2007) *Insight Dialogue: The interpersonal path to freedom.* Boulder, CO: Shambhala Publications, p.22.

3   Kramer, G. (2007) *Insight Dialogue: The interpersonal path to freedom.* Boulder, CO: Shambhala Publications, p.29.

4   Smith, H., and Novak, P. (2003) *Buddhism: A concise introduction.* New York: Harper San Francisco.

5   Kramer, G. (2007) *Insight Dialogue: The interpersonal path to freedom.* Boulder, CO: Shambhala Publications, pp.76–77.

6   Gethin, R. (1998) *The Foundations of Buddhism.* Oxford: Oxford University Press, pp.81–82.

7   Gunaratana, B. (2001) *Eight Mindful Steps to Happiness.* Somerville, MA: Wisdom Publications.

8   Kramer, G. (2020) *A Whole-Life Path.* Seattle, WA: Insight Dialogue Community.

— Chapter 8 —

OPENING THE COMPASSIONATE HEART

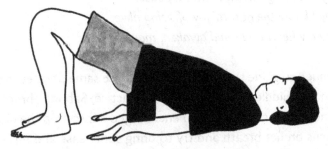

Supported Bridge is a gentle backbend that can open the heart-space to allow compassion in

About one year after I started teaching lovingkindness practices to my talk therapy clients and yoga therapy clients and interweaving them into many of my yin yoga classes, many people reported that they felt more gentle, loving, and compassionate toward themselves and others in their lives. The first time one of my clients had an abreaction (an overwhelming emotional response to a situation that brings back painful memories from a previous traumatic event) to a lovingkindness practice was in the inpatient setting I worked in. The yoga therapy group was made up of six clients with different emotional and cognitive challenges.

One client, Sabrina, was really enjoying the group and stated that her depression and anxiety had decreased significantly since she had started the sessions four weeks earlier. In the earlier sessions, Sabrina was able to meditate and do gentle yoga without any significant challenges and would often practice on her own following the group sessions.

This week, I could see right away that something was different. As I described the purpose of lovingkindness practices which included a guided meditation to offer phrases of care in turn to oneself, a dear loved one, a neutral person, and a challenging person, Sabrina's eyes looked angry. She said, "This seems stupid." I invited her and the group to make space for themselves to include both positive and negative feelings that might come up during the practice. I suggested that even if they did not immediately feel compassionate toward themselves or others, their willingness to try to connect and open their hearts was the first step toward lovingkindness. I began the practice and invited participants to offer phrases of lovingkindness to themselves that were suggested by one of my teachers, Tara Brach:

> *May I be filled with lovingkindness; may I be held in lovingkindness.*
> *May I accept myself just as I am.*
> *May I be happy.*
> *May I touch great and natural peace.*
> *May I know the natural joy of being alive.*
> *May my heart and mind awaken; may I be free.*[1]

I continued to guide the clients to offer these same phrases to someone they love. In the middle of this part of the practice, Sabrina abruptly opened her eyes and said, "I can't do this." I encouraged her to stop the practice for now and focus on her breath and try to bring some ease and relaxation into her body. She would not have it, or any other suggestions I was offering.

She started to cry loudly, and I paused the group and took her outside the room to process what was happening. She stated that no one loved her and that she felt like this practice only highlighted her intense loneliness. She felt left out and rejected by the practice and very angry at me because I should have known about her past family trauma and how depressed she was. I sat with her as she became more and more tearful and upset, but holding space for her did not seem to be helping. Instead, I suggested we practice one more time together with a different focus.

"What if we could offer these phrases of care to the planet—to plants, animals, and people all over the world?"

She hesitated and then nodded slowly. "Okay, let's try this."

We sat and breathed together. This time, I asked her to imagine offering prayers of well-being and good wishes to all beings everywhere. Again, using Tara Brach's beautiful phrases, I said, "May all beings be filled with loving-kindness. May all beings know great and natural peace. May there be peace on earth, peace everywhere. May all beings awaken; may all be free."

Sabrina began to relax, and I saw her breath deepen as we got to the final phrase. We sat together for a few minutes in silence. Her eyes were soft and damp. She said that she could feel her heart now. That is the power of these heart practices, even when people have significant wounding of the heart.

THE FOUR HEART QUALITIES: LOVINGKINDNESS, COMPASSION, EMPATHETIC JOY, AND EQUANIMITY

Infusing the Eightfold Path, described in the last chapter, are the *brahma-viharas* in the Pali language. They are referred to as *the four immeasurables, the four radiant abodes,* or *the four heart qualities.* They include lovingkindness, compassion, empathetic joy, and equanimity. These qualities serve to dissolve the boundaries that create separateness and isolation, so we can deepen our connection with others. In addition, these four qualities can be cultivated as a meditation path that can foster deeper and more sustained states of concentration leading to wisdom. Jack Kornfield, author and international teacher of Buddhism in the West, writes:

> These abodes are the expression of natural human happiness. They are immediate and simple, the universal description of an open heart. Even when we hear their names—love, compassion, joy, peace—they touch us directly. When we meet another who is filled with these qualities, our heart lights up. When we touch peace, love, joy, and compassion in ourselves, we are transformed.[2]

In my many years of meditation training and practice, I found that these teachings around the four heart qualities have been the most transformational part of my meditation journey. They speak to me in their simplicity around opening the heart and connecting to others with compassion and love. Over and over again, when I am struggling to find inner kindness or am feeling angry and gripped by some hurt or wound, I return to the teachings around the four heart qualities. They have a profound effect on me almost immediately, like a soothing balm or calm warm breeze, and I find that my constricted heart begins to open again.

The Buddhist path describes specific practices to strengthen our capacity to experience and cultivate these four qualities. While we may possess these qualities as part of our innate goodness, all of us need practices to keep the heart open and balanced, especially during difficult times, on an internal and external level. These practices are part of a meditation path and include specific guided reflections, intentions, and repetition of phrases that can open the heart; if done regularly, they do open the heart and create a sense of connection and harmony.

Each of the four qualities can be seen as a continuum from wholesome to unwholesome. Jack Kornfield states that wholesome qualities are coming from an awakened heart (love, compassion, empathetic joy, and equanimity). "Near enemies," in contrast, are qualities that may look similar to the pure qualities of the heart but can actually cause a feeling of disconnection or separateness. Finally, he explains that "far enemies" are on the opposite side of the continuum from the wholesome qualities as they can cause harm or close the heart.[3] Because this continuum can be subtle, it is helpful to consider an example.

Lovingkindness is a wholesome quality. However, when someone has an unhealthy or conditional attachment to another person (e.g., "I will love you as long as you are there for me"), that same quality becomes the near enemy because it can cause clinging and fear. On the opposite side of the spectrum— the far enemy—is hatred, which produces harm and causes suffering whenever it is directed at someone.

Part of the meditation practice is to be able to identify and nourish the wholesome qualities and reduce or eliminate the near and far enemies. It is difficult for the mind to actually hold a wholesome quality like lovingkindness and a far enemy like hatred at the same time. So, the four qualities act as antidotes for corresponding harmful qualities, essentially counteracting our negative thoughts or intentions by introducing and cultivating positive intentions or thoughts. From a neuroscience perspective, this stimulation of positive thoughts occurs in one part of the brain while effectively quieting parts of the brain that are responsible for fear or anger. Author Rick Hanson, in his instructive book *Buddha's Brain*, describes this process as "reciprocal inhibition."[4] When we utilize meditative practices to enhance the four heart qualities, we can actually change how we think! Hanson describes it this way: "What flows through your mind sculpts your brain. Thus, you can use your mind to change your brain for the better—which will benefit your whole being and every other person whose life you touch."[5]

LOVINGKINDNESS

The first heart quality, lovingkindness, or *metta* in the Pali language of the Buddha, is considered the foundation for the other qualities. This type of love is different from the passion or attachment types of love we often think about when we hear this word. In Buddhist teachings, lovingkindness is a sense of openness, warmth, and care that is not dependent on another person. Long-time mindfulness teacher Sharon Salzberg describes this quality in her book

Lovingkindness: The Revolutionary Art of Happiness: "Metta—the sense of love that is not bound to desire, that does not have to pretend that things are other than the way they are—overcomes the illusion of separateness, of not being part of the whole."[6] By practicing lovingkindness toward oneself and others, the suffering that so many of us experience by feeling unloved, disconnected, and alone begins to ease. The beginning of this practice for new students often involves the recognition that we wish to be happy and that others have this same basic wish. By starting with this very simple premise, we can begin to move past the suffering many people experience around feeling undeserving of love or kindness and move toward a basic understanding that humans want to be happy and find ease and connection. Salzberg writes:

> Looking at people and communicating that they can be loved, and they can love in return, is giving them a tremendous gift. It is also a gift to ourselves. We see that we are one with the fabric of life. This is the power of *metta*: to teach ourselves and the world this inherent loveliness.[7]

Lovingkindness (and its near and far enemies of attachment and hatred) shows up in all our daily activities, in how we take care of ourselves each day, our self-talk, how we view others when we greet them or scroll through social media, and certainly in our yoga practice. Yin yoga invites us—right from the very beginning when we take our first pose—to consider practicing lovingkindness. Yin yoga is a practice of lovingkindness achieved by cultivating space and ease in the body, mind, and heart. Yin invites us to meet our experiences with kindness even when strong sensations arise that might be difficult to stay with. As we stay in a pose for several minutes, when uncomfortable sensations arise, lovingkindness can help us to stay in the pose as we learn how to intentionally cultivate presence and care for ourselves. When I am practicing yin, I will often infuse my poses with a specific intention or wish for inner and outer happiness such as the ones described below:

May I be happy.
May I find ease and space.
May I accept myself just as I am.
May I be free from inner or outer pain.

Because yin yoga is a less active and muscularly engaged practice than many forms of Hatha yoga, we are more easily able to let go of attachments and outcomes (e.g., weight loss, mastering a peak pose), and our grasping for perfection as yoga students. While we still may want to work toward increasing our flexibility or openness, the competitive nature of some Hatha yoga practices is eliminated with yin. Attachment (the near enemy to lovingkindness) can create suffering. As we learn how to relax and stay with the sensations of breath, we can ease further away from the far enemies of lovingkindness, including fear, anger, and hatred. Finally, in the space of holding yin poses, we can begin to cultivate lovingkindness for others by recognizing that we are not alone. Our experiences in this moment (even our discomfort) are natural and part of living in a body.

Just as we would like to experience ease and happiness, we can recognize that the student next to us in class feels the same basic needs and desires. To generate lovingkindness toward others, we might imagine certain people and offer them gentle wishes of care:

May you be happy.
May you find ease and space.
May you accept yourself just as you are.
May you be free from inner or outer pain.

By wishing others ease and happiness, many of us will experience a warmth inside of ourselves. This warmth of connection is at the heart of lovingkindness: unconditional friendliness. These moments of genuine connection with others and ourselves help us to directly experience what it feels like to be openhearted. In Western society, where there is so much emphasis on doing, achieving, earning, and creating, these simple practices remind us of our basic humanity. Alan B. Wallace, Buddhist scholar, writes in his book *Genuine Happiness,* "We come to relate to ourselves with gentle, nonjudgmental acceptance, and we extend this loving heart to all those around us, who, like ourselves, wish to find happiness."[8]

COMPASSION

Compassion, the second of the four heart qualities, is at the very root of Buddhism and many other religions. Compassion, or *karuna* in Pali, is defined as a wish for others to be free from suffering. Mindfulness teacher and clinical psychologist Tara Brach's writings around compassion have helped to bring a contemporary psychological perspective to these wisdom teachings. She writes in her book *Radical Acceptance*:

Classical Buddhist texts describe compassion as the quivering of the heart, a visceral tenderness in the face of suffering. In the Buddhist tradition, one who has realized the fullness of compassion and lives from compassion is called a *bodhisattva*. The *bodhisattva*'s path and teaching are that when we allow our hearts to be touched by suffering—our own or another's—our natural compassion flowers.[9]

Compassion helps us to recognize and care about the suffering of others. The Dalai Lama, in his book *The Art of Happiness*, describes compassion as "a state of mind that is nonviolent, nonharming, and nonaggressive. It is a mental attitude based on the wish for others to be free of their suffering and is associated with a sense of commitment, responsibility, and respect toward the other."[10] We can find a shared humanity in this basic understanding that we as humans do not want to suffer, just as we can find joy in the understanding that we want to be happy. Our yin yoga practice can assist us in generating compassion both for ourselves and for others. When we first meet uncomfortable sensations in a yin pose or experience feelings that are painful, many of us will appraise these experiences as "negative," "difficult," or even as a kind of suffering. This appraisal will often lead to aversion or trying to move away from the moment.

I have had this experience many times during my yin practice, particularly in poses where the sensations are strongest (Saddle, Dragon). My first reaction is usually "get me out of here," which creates very little opportunity for curiosity or exploration. However, by focusing on compassion, we can begin to turn toward the sensation and acknowledge that while this may be uncomfortable, we can "be with it" or be "with ourselves." Further, we have complete choice about whether to stay in the pose, modify, prop, or simply come out of it and find an alternative. We have effectively moved away from suffering and the aversion that can result and moved toward compassionate and wise action.

If we begin to feel sorry for ourselves (the near enemy of compassion, which is pity or despair), we are more likely to give up and not let ourselves experience what the pose or corresponding feeling has to reveal to us. If we become very agitated or physically uncomfortable, we may even become angry or turn on ourselves or our practice (this is the far enemy of compassion: hatred or cruelty) and give ourselves extremely negative messages about something being wrong with us, with the teacher, or with the practice. To soften into compassion in yin, I will often invite the following expressions:

I can be with this sensation for now.
Yes, this is hard.
I am willing to meet myself here.
I can stay here for five more breaths.

I love practicing yin in a group format because we have a sense of community and that we are not alone in our challenging experiences. We might even begin to offer compassion to others in the room.

> *May you experience freedom from suffering.*
> *I am here with you.*
> *We are all in this together.*

In *The Art of Happiness: A Handbook for Living,* the Dalai Lama writes:

> In the same way that physical pain unifies our sense of having a body, we can conceive of the general experience of suffering acting as a unifying force that connects us with others. Perhaps it is the ultimate meaning behind our suffering. It is our suffering that is the most basic element that we share with others, the factor that unifies us with all living creatures.[11]

In our yin practice, we can intentionally cultivate physical discomfort, yet rather than feeling victimized or alone, we can also intentionally cultivate compassion toward ourselves and others, allowing our yoga to become a practice field for opening the heart over and over.

EMPATHETIC JOY

Empathetic or vicarious joy, or *mudita* in Pali, refers to the ability to rejoice in the happiness of another. Alan Wallace, author and expert on Tibetan Buddhism, says, "Once you have begun to develop the first two of the Four Immeasurables—lovingkindness and compassion—you will find that empathetic joy and equanimity come quite naturally."[12] This type of joy has an openhearted quality that comes from feeling so connected to another person that we celebrate their happiness as if it were our own. This type of joy is different from a more grasping and fleeting quality of joy that occurs when we receive praise from our boss or buy a new car—that good feeling that starts to ebb away as soon as the new car smell wears off or our boss makes a negative comment to us. Empathetic joy has an open quality that is not shallow like a Facebook "like" on a photo we've posted or happiness over our own personal gains and successes (these are the near enemies, frivolity and hypocrisy). Empathetic joy has an embodied quality that can be felt in the heart.

Expressions like "warm heart" and "heart singing" offer us a description of the felt sense of empathetic joy. Like the other heart qualities, we are naturally born with openness and joy. Whenever we observe children, we see a natural, joyful quality in how they laugh, play, and smile. Often this joy fades as children reach the stormy teenage years or experience traumas during their foundational developmental periods. However, we can cultivate joy through our practices to open the heart. In our yin practice, the cultivation of empathetic joy starts with the practice of embodiment. Coming into a shape, we can begin to observe the sensations directly in the body. As we stay connected in the pose, more and more subtle observations in the body can be felt, including any barriers that we may be experiencing that might lead us into the far enemies of joy, including self-preoccupied negativity, envy, or hopelessness. If the heart feels closed off in some way, we can begin to explore ways to soften and open it by first acknowledging how our beliefs or feelings may be limiting our capacity for joy. From here, we can begin to focus on a sensation in the body that we appreciate (I often like to focus on a neutral area like my hands or feet) and pause to savor that experience. That begins turning us toward a more embodied or natural sense of joy. Once more, I like to introduce phrases that can support this journey toward embodied joy while in a pose:

> *I can hold space for my _____ [pain, depression, judgment].*
> *I can say yes to my experience as it is.*
> *I am grateful for my legs that allow me to feel the ground beneath me.*
> *My heart is open and full.*
> *May others be happy and know the natural joy of being alive.*

During each pose, I invite a similar investigation of the places that feel shut down or restricted and then a slow turning toward these places with compassion; this is followed by directing attention toward those sensations that are open, free, and spacious. By the end of a yin series, we have practiced turning toward joy and openness over and over again with the changing conditions of each pose.

EQUANIMITY

The fourth heart quality, equanimity or *upekha*, is perhaps the most challenging to both understand and inhabit. The traditional definition in Buddhism is *even-mindedness* or *impartiality*. However, this can be easily misunderstood to mean *detachment* or *indifference* (near enemies of equanimity). Alan Wallace describes it like this:

The inner quality to be cultivated here is more than a feeling; it is a stance, an attitude—a way of attending to others that involves neither attachment to those who are near, nor aversion to anyone who might impede our happiness. So, equanimity—in the context of the Four Immeasurables—balances our perspective on others. We transcend attachment and aversion, attaining a sense of even-mindedness. This is based simply on the recognition that every sentient being, human and otherwise, is like ourselves, seeking happiness, wishing to be free of suffering.[13]

The other three heart qualities of lovingkindness, compassion, and joy rely on the foundation of equanimity, including being present, openhearted, and able to respond with a heart-opening feeling toward others. So, if we see someone struggling with a painful emotion like anger or grief, we can acknowledge that we, too, suffer from the same afflictions and we can share our concern for that person and wish for them to be free from suffering. Alan Wallace says:

Develop this even concern, even loving-kindness, even compassion, the even caring for others, regardless of their conduct. This kind of equanimity is indispensable. Without it, love, compassion, and empathetic joy will always be conditional, tainted by self-centered attachment. So, equanimity, this impartiality, is an essential component of the Four Immeasurables.[14]

The far enemy or tainted version of equanimity is seeing others as the enemy or the "other," which can lead to prejudice and even repulsion. Equanimity is the antidote to discrimination and hatred, which is, in large part, what ails our world today. In yin yoga, we are inviting an attitude of equanimity in each pose at the very foundation of our practice. When I am focusing on this quality in my teaching, I begin by asking my students to start exactly where they are. I will cue them with the simple inquiry question: *What is happening now?* This inquiry allows students to be fully present, awake, and reflective. The responses might include a physical sensation, a thought, a feeling, or an emotion. At this point, I recommend utilizing phrases while in the postures to support this sense of space and balance:

May I be balanced.
May I find peace and ease.
May I be open.

As students move into the next pose, I have them notice what has changed, again using the simple inquiry: *What is happening now?* As students key into what has already come and gone and what is occurring right now, it is important to enter into understanding that all things come and go over time and to connect to the bigger picture outside of ourselves. I recommend including the following phrases:

> *May I learn to see the changing nature of all things with equanimity and balance.*
> *May I bring compassion and equanimity to those in need.*

Finally, I suggest in the latter part of the practice allowing students to remain in silence and stay with this open presence. I suggest a practice that Jack Kornfield calls A Mind Like Sky meditation. He says:

> In this circumstance we can open the lens of attention to its widest angle and let our awareness become like space or the sky. As the Buddha instructs in the Majjhima Nikaya, "Develop a mind that is vast like space, where experiences both pleasant and unpleasant can appear and disappear without conflict, struggle or harm. Rest in a mind like vast sky."[15]

ENDNOTES

1 Brach, T. (2004) *Radical Acceptance: Embracing your life with the heart of a Buddha.* New York: Bantam Books, pp.278–279.
2 Kornfield, J. (2011) *Bringing Home the Dharma.* Boulder, CO: Shambhala Publications, p.25.
3 Kornfield, J. (2011) *Bringing Home the Dharma.* Boulder, CO: Shambhala Publications.
4 Hanson, R., and Mendius, R. (2009) *Buddha's Brain: The practical neuroscience of happiness, love and wisdom.* Oakland, CA: New Harbinger Publications, p.186.
5 Hanson, R., and Mendius, R. (2009) *Buddha's Brain: The practical neuroscience of happiness, love and wisdom.* Oakland, CA: New Harbinger Publications, p.6.
6 Salzberg, S. (1995) *Lovingkindness: The revolutionary art of happiness.* Boston, MA: Shambhala Publications, p.21.
7 Salzberg, S. (1995) *Lovingkindness: The revolutionary art of happiness.* Boston, MA: Shambhala Publications, p.28.
8 Wallace, B.A. (2005) *Genuine Happiness.* Hoboken, NJ: John Wiley & Sons, p.122.
9 Brach, T. (2003) *Radical Acceptance.* New York: Bantam Books, p.200.
10 Dalai Lama XIV, and Cutler, H. (1998) *The Art of Happiness: A handbook for living.* New York: Riverhead Books, p.114.
11 Dalai Lama XIV, and Cutler, H. (1998) *The Art of Happiness: A handbook for living.* New York: Riverhead Books, p.206.
12 Wallace, B.A. (2005) *Genuine Happiness.* Hoboken, NJ: John Wiley & Sons, p.129.
13 Wallace, B.A. (2005) *Genuine Happiness.* Hoboken, NJ: John Wiley & Sons, p.149.
14 Wallace, B.A. (2005) *Genuine Happiness.* Hoboken, NJ: John Wiley & Sons, p.150.
15 Kornfield, J. (2021) 'A Mind Like Sky meditation.' https://jackkornfield.com/a-mind-like-sky.

— Chapter 9 —

TURNING WITHIN

Yin Yoga and Psychology

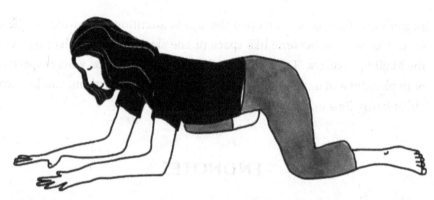

Frog can help us practice self-soothing when we are at the edge of our comfort zone

My yoga therapy client, Rachel, came into our session with a worried expression on her face. She shared that she was feeling overwhelmed by the demands of school (she was a first-year law student at an extremely competitive program) and was struggling with insomnia and difficulty concentrating.

As we moved through a series of warm-ups, she appeared distracted and uncomfortable. I suggested that she choose a yin posture where she could stay for a while without effort or trying to accomplish anything. She selected Butterfly and I took time to cover her with a blanket and place blocks underneath her knees to provide additional support. I guided her through a brief meditation and asked if she would be comfortable to speak out loud at times during the practice as a part of a spoken inquiry practice. She agreed and as we moved through grounding, breathing, and body scan, her body relaxed, and her breathing began to settle. I asked her to notice "What is arising in this moment?"

Her breathing began to speed up again, and she reported, "I am having worried thoughts." I responded, "Tell me more about that." She shared, "If I don't do well on my exams this semester, I won't be asked to do law review next year. If I am not on law review, I will blow my chances of getting a job in a good law firm. If I don't get a good job, I will have mounds of student debt that I can't pay back, and I won't be able to get married and start a family."

Rachel began to cry softly as she got to this last part. I asked her, "Is there anything else arising in this moment?" In a very quiet voice she responded, "I never measure up. I am a disappointment." As I took in her words, my first instinct was to reassure her that she was extremely competent, intelligent, and far from a disappointment. However, part of the yin yoga journey is for Rachel to be able to observe and hold the truth of her experience just as it is. I asked her if there was an image or sensation (hard, heavy, fluttery, spacious) that came with this feeling of disappointment, and she was able to share that she noticed "a huge hole in my stomach that feels empty and dark."

I then asked her if she would be willing to try an experiment with me. She nodded and I invited her to consider the opposite of disappointment. "Reflect on a time when you felt successful, competent, and strong. Is there an image or sensation that comes up as you consider this feeling?"

Rachel shared that she felt "strong and determined intensity hard and deep in my solar plexus." I invited her stay with that sensation for a while. Then I asked her to locate the opposite, "the disappointment," again in her body. I had her move back and forth a few times between both sensations. I asked her if she would be able to hold both experiences at the same time.

She quietly remained in her yin posture, and I could see her body become more and more relaxed. I asked her if there was a belief that was associated with the feeling of disappointment and she responded, "I sometimes feel like I am not good enough." I asked her again to move through a series of reflections. First, to identify if there was a sensation that accompanied this belief. Then, if there was a sensation, to locate it in the body. She identified a sharp pain in her belly. If possible, I instructed, find an opposite to this belief. She said, "I am good enough."

I asked her to notice where a sensation associated with this opposite was felt in the body. She indicated that she felt her heart soften. Once again, I instructed her to hold both sensations at the same time. I asked her if there was something that she would like to say to these two beliefs, "I am not good enough" and "I am good enough." She said quietly, "Even though I doubt myself, I recognize that I am good enough."

I had Rachel transition into a simple Reclining Twist and had her continue to work with this emerging skill to hold both her doubt and her core belief about her goodness as she allowed her body to settle into the next shape. By the time she came to the second side of the twist, her belief had changed again, and she was left with simply "I am good enough."

In her yin practice, Rachel demonstrated some of the potent effects of cognitive-behavioral techniques within a yin yoga session. She was able to identify and stay with the sensations in her body as she explored her automatic negative thoughts. Once she identified her core negative belief, she was able to work with opposites and discovered a powerful positive core belief to strengthen her self-identity. The yin poses provided her with a safe, quiet, and stable place to do this interior work.

Cognitive behavioral therapies (CBT) are a popular, evidence-based, and well-regarded type of psychotherapy treatment that share some basic underlying principles and features. Pioneered by Aaron Beck in 1970, CBT's core premise is that *negative or maladaptive cognitions* that are faulty or distorted in some way can cause psychological distress, including negative emotions and maladaptive behaviors. In Beck's model, "these maladaptive cognitions include general beliefs, or schemas, about the world, the self, and the future, giving rise to specific and automatic thoughts in particular situations."[1] CBT is one of the most common orientations for practicing psychologists because of its relatively structured approach using treatment protocols that can be easily administered and replicated; this has resulted in a large research base with impressive outcomes for many emotional disorders in children, adolescents, and adults.[2]

CBT typically involves helping the client to identify maladaptive beliefs or thoughts, evaluate them for possible distortions, and then modify them based on more realistic, positive, and adaptive cognitions. Thinking about a particular event, person, or situation, which can be described as *subjective cognitive appraisal*, is the key mechanism of action and change in CBT treatment. Categories of popular CBT treatments include traditional cognitive therapy, dialectical behavioral therapy (DBT), mindfulness-based cognitive therapy, schema-focused therapy, and acceptance and commitment therapy.

Current CBT treatments often combine a variety of different modalities, such as mindfulness, positive behavioral supports, and physiological or body-based interventions. These *hybrid* CBT treatments are often referred to as the "third wave" or next generation of CBT, with the use of new methods for addressing faulty beliefs or negative thoughts, including the emphasis on acceptance of one's thoughts rather than trying to control them, reducing stress in the body to find more ease in the mind, and utilizing effective coping skills when emotions are heightened.[3] Research indicates that a number of psychological conditions

can be treated effectively using these hybrid CBT treatments, including anxiety disorders, eating disorders, anger management, somatoform disorders,
and stress.[4]

One of the most common criticisms of CBT typically centers around the fact
that the treatment can seem highly mechanistic with its reliance on protocols
and scripts to change faulty cognitions rather than focusing on the whole person
or what is unique about their story. Other criticisms center around the lack of
neuroscientific evidence to demonstrate the efficacy of treatment outside the
therapy setting in actual clinical laboratories.[5]

In my own practice as a psychologist, I have found the first criticism around
the mechanistic aspect of CBT and its over-reliance on changing thoughts over
other important humanistic considerations to be accurate in many respects.
When emphasizing cognition and using "talk therapy" only to reflect on the
cognition, I found myself curious what else might be happening for the person
sitting in front of me. There were often incongruent moments where their
words did not match their physical presentation. For example, one of my clients,
Beth, was speaking about her belief that she was not a good enough mother to
her disabled daughter. Her voice was calm, and she was able to discuss these
beliefs with an openness and candor that to most observers would indicate
that she was comfortable exploring these topics. However, her subtle body
language, including the tightening of her fists, a downturned facial expression,
and slumped shoulders, indicated something much more intense.

When I asked her to notice "What is happening in the body right now as you
share this?" she again used measured, calm speech and said, "Not much." She
described how she was aware of her own beliefs and that they did not surprise
her in the least. I invited her to close her eyes and come into a gentle meditation
seat. I asked her to silently visualize where in her body she experienced that core
belief "Not a good enough mother."

She took a long time before nodding and agreeing to explore in her body.
Within a few minutes, I observed a softening in her facial features, and tears
began to stream down her cheeks. I gently asked her to stay with the sensations
in her body without having to say or do anything. For the next few minutes,
she cried softly, and her breath began to slow down. Her posture relaxed and
her facial expression shifted.

I asked her to share what had happened when she was ready, and she said,
"I was stuck in my head and felt cut off from my body. I had no idea that there
was so much grief and shame inside of me." We were able to use some of the
compassion practices described in Chapter 8 to help her nourish and gently
calm her nervous system. By inviting the body to provide feedback, she was able

to integrate some of the distress that her core beliefs were causing her while at the same time bypassing some of the defenses and barriers that her mind was creating. Further, she was also beginning to create skills to work with distressing or charged emotions through the doorway of the body, truly operating from a mind-body integrative approach. Like Beth, many of my clients can get stuck when they stay focused on their thoughts. Many of these thoughts are negative and are linked to stories about the past that continue to serve as reminders about what is wrong with them, others, or the world around them.

By creating a doorway to the body, we can help clients move out of the repetitive cycle of thinking and explore current and present-moment experiences in the body. Yin yoga can serve as a vehicle to bridge this mind-body connection. By using CBT strategies coupled with the direct sensations that yin poses provide, I have a systematic but gentle approach to helping clients move toward self-determination in accessing and processing their feelings that come from deeply held beliefs.

There are three CBT approaches that I find particularly helpful to utilize in conjunction with yin yoga when I'm working with clients who have core beliefs or negative thoughts rooted in early childhood experiences and the ensuing painful emotions that occur when they are stuck in recursive thought patterns. These approaches are dialectical behavioral therapy (DBT), working with automatic negative thoughts (ANTs, which will be described below), and Internal Family Systems (IFS). It is important to note that these are powerful techniques that should not be used without specific training in psychotherapy. Further, I strongly recommend setting up supervision with a licensed clinician, especially in the beginning stages of using these techniques, and ensuring that one has a client's full consent indicating that they understand the risks and benefits of using such psychological techniques prior to starting treatment.

As I describe the use of these psychological models in a yin practice, I am doing so as both a licensed psychologist and a yoga therapist. Some of the techniques can be utilized in a group setting as they are sufficiently broad and applicable to many people. However, the yoga guide must be aware that they can evoke strong emotions and may prefer to utilize only a select group of skills that provide an introduction to inner work. I will often suggest to my yoga students after a class where I have introduced a concept like automatic negative thoughts that they may want to consider going to a licensed clinical therapist if they would like to explore these ideas on a deeper level.

AUTOMATIC NEGATIVE THOUGHTS

Changing maladaptive thought patterns are at the very heart of CBT approaches. One of the models that I have found to be very helpful in terms of its simplicity, practicability, and ease of use is the concept of working with automatic negative thoughts. Daniel Amen, MD, describes automatic negative thoughts as "cynical, gloomy, and complaining thoughts that just seem to keep marching in all by themselves."[6] He describes nine different types of ANTs that can interfere with well-being and lead to depression and anxiety. These include:

- "All or nothing" thinking: Examples might be: "I'll never get a promotion," or "My husband always seems unhappy." Using absolute terms like "never" and "always" can lead to strong activation in the limbic system.
- Focusing on the negative: We looked at the negativity bias in Chapter 5 regarding negative emotions, and this comes up again here in terms of the frequency of negative thoughts. An example is focusing on the one negative comment in a performance review.
- Fortune-telling: This relates to predicting outcomes (almost always negative). Examples might include "I know I am going to fail this exam," "I am sure that this relationship will not work out in the end."
- Mind reading: This comes up in interpersonal relations where you believe (falsely) that you know what the other person is thinking or feeling. Examples might include "You are mad at me, I can tell," or "I know you don't really want to go on this trip."
- Thinking with your feelings: This creates a sense of certitude that your feelings are *fact* rather than just *feelings*. Examples might include "I feel like a complete failure," or "I feel like nobody will ever love me."
- Guilt beating: The evocation of guilt can be extremely painful when it is another person blaming us for something and even more wounding when we beat ourselves up when something goes wrong. Examples might be "I should have tried harder to make the relationship work," or "It is my fault that I am having money problems."
- Labeling: When we label ourselves or others, we are often using a quick, easily recognized name that captures a feeling. However, this habit short-changes the complexity of the person, situation, or condition and is often mean-spirited. Examples: "She is irresponsible," or "I am a complete idiot."
- Personalizing: This occurs when we construct a story that involves our

own personal role in a situation. Examples: "My friend did not text me back so she must be mad at me," or "My daughter got in a car accident because I didn't stop her from driving in the dark."

- Blaming: This last ANT is the most harmful, according to Daniel Amen. He describes it as "the most poisonous red ant"[7] because it creates a sense of powerlessness and victimization which can make it very difficult to find the motivation to change the situation. Many relationships are ruined when partners turn on each other in this way. Examples: "You make my life miserable," or "It's your fault that I am so unhappy."

When I work with clients who are struggling with ANTs (and frankly, most of us struggle with them), I use a series of inquiry questions to help work with the thoughts. Many of my clients want their ANTs to go away, but it is important to recognize that we need to engage with our thoughts to make changes rather than trying to make them go away.

First, it is important to identify the thoughts. Many people do not even realize that they are continually responding to this internal dialogue of thoughts through their beliefs, emotions, and actions. So, I recommend tracking the ANTs we say to ourselves for a few days to get a sense of the common ones that are operating without our even recognizing them. This is actually the most important step, because as soon as we make conscious the thoughts that were operating beneath our awareness, we loosen their grip on us. I particularly like the term ANT because it allows us to take these thoughts less seriously. Once we recognize them as ANTs, we have the freedom to actually work with them.

This series of inquiry areas allows us to bring ANTs out into the open where we can challenge them:

FIRST INQUIRY AREA: IDENTIFYING THE ANTS

- What ANTs are present right now?
- Are these repetitive?
- When do they come out?

SECOND INQUIRY AREA: IMPACT OF THE ANTS

- How do your ANTs affect your mood?

- How does your body feel?

THIRD INQUIRY AREA: EXAMINE THE MESSAGE

One of the challenges around working with thoughts is that we believe them! Sages and writers over the millennia from the Buddha to Mark Twain to Eckhart Tolle have encouraged us not to believe our thoughts. They recognized that believing our thoughts often leads to suffering. They understood that our thoughts don't tell the complete truth and sometimes even lie to us! By asking ourselves the following inquiry questions, we can begin to look at our thoughts more compassionately, further loosening their emotional grip on us.

- Is this thought truthful?
- Is this thought helpful or harmful?

FOURTH INQUIRY AREA: CHALLENGE THE ANTS

Once you have identified the ANTs and examined the messages, it is time to challenge them. Through repeatedly challenging them, you can train your thoughts to be more positive. Here are two examples of ways to compassionately challenge your negative thoughts.

- What would you tell a loved one or friend if they shared this negative thought with you?
- What is the opposite of this negative thought?

In Yin yoga, we are often confronted by ANTs from the moment we take our first pose. A few of my favorite ANTs from my own practice include "I hate yin yoga" (seriously, I have said this), "My yoga practice is pathetic," "I am too fat to do this pose," and on and on. In the quietude of a yin pose, I will often ask students to begin tracking, observing the subtle and more overt negative messages that they are sending to themselves.

One of the most helpful experiences in working with negative thoughts is to actually have the direct felt experience that they are incorrect. For example, "I am too fat to do this pose" may come up for students, like it did for me. Then, once a student can settle into the pose, find the shape that is most appropriate for their body, and find some ease, they can challenge the thought with a more truthful and compassionate expression. "My body is ____ [strong, open, flexible, alive] in this pose." I have students that have told me in yin class that they have enjoyed yoga for the first time because they were actually able to do all of the poses offered. Many of them had ANTs that were present during their yoga practice in the past but they were able to challenge those thoughts through their direct experience. Yin yoga can be used to work with ANTs whether they directly relate to the practice in that moment or they are a pattern of negative thoughts that are accompanying the student to the class. Being prepared to meet negative thoughts, especially when we are in a quiet practice such as yin, can take us from believing the thoughts or trying to push them away, to turning toward them using inquiry in the practice itself, and recognizing that this can be part of the practice rather than interference.

DIALECTICAL BEHAVIOR THERAPY

Dialectical behavior therapy (DBT) is considered the gold standard of CBT treatment for clients with borderline personality disorder (BPD), who frequently engage in suicidal or self-injurious behaviors. Developed by Marsha Linehan, DBT integrates principles from behavioral therapy, gestalt therapy, cognitive behavioral therapy, humanistic client-centered therapy, and mindfulness. DBT offers a practical, skills-based model for clients in both individual and group formats.[8, 9]

The term *dialectical* is shorthand for "an overarching dialectical worldview that emphasizes the synthesis of opposites."[10] In addition, *dialectical* refers to the "multiple tensions that co-occur in therapy with suicidal clients with BPD as well as the emphasis in DBT of enhancing dialectical thinking patterns to replace rigid dichotomous thinking."[11] By using mindfulness and other methods of validation, DBT can help clients to accept their current difficulties while at the same time allowing them to learn skills that will help them cope in more adaptive, less destructive ways. To develop the skill of acceptance in DBT, one must utilize mindfulness to become aware of thoughts, feelings, emotions, and physical sensations while at the same time learning not to judge or criticize oneself, others, or the experience. This skill, coined *radical acceptance* by Marsha Linehan, reflects the importance of releasing the harsh judgments that often lead to more suffering and distress in order to begin healing.[12, 13]

In the first of four stages of DBT, the main focus is on helping clients to reduce extreme, even life-threatening behaviors—including suicidal ideation and threats of violence and self-harm—through the development of skills to stabilize and improve overall behavioral control through the following pathways:

emotion regulation, or improving the capacity to regulate extreme emotions; *distress tolerance,* or tolerating a range of feelings; *interpersonal effectiveness,* or developing improved communication skills; *mindfulness*, or maintaining a heightened and nonjudgmental self-awareness in the moment; and *self-management* or better self-control.

Stages two through four of DBT are focused on quality of life and well-being. "In the subsequent stages, the treatment goals are to replace 'quiet desperation' with non-traumatic emotional experiencing [stage 2], to achieve 'ordinary' happiness and unhappiness and reduce ongoing disorders and problems in living [stage 3], and to resolve a sense of incompleteness and achieve joy [stage 4]."[14]

I do not recommend utilizing a DBT approach without sufficient training as a licensed mental health professional, background in the DBT model, and supervision with a trained DBT professional. I have received extensive training in DBT as a psychologist and have utilized these skills in multiple formats, including traditional DBT skills groups and individual psychotherapy as well as integrating them into yoga therapy. Many clients have told me that having these skills to fall back on during times of stress, emotional upheaval, or physical distress has been a vital part of their ability to navigate difficult times. DBT can be used in conjunction with yin yoga to address naturally evoked uncomfortable sensations, emotions, and thoughts that arise.

In Table 9.1, I provide examples of DBT skills in each of the four modules described above: emotion regulation, distress tolerance, interpersonal effectiveness, and mindfulness. The specific DBT practices are described in depth in Part 2. In brief, they are:

> **REST:** relax; evaluate; set an intention; take action
> **Radical acceptance:** stop fighting reality
> **Wise Mind:** the balance between reason and emotion
> **ABC PLEASE:** ABC—accumulate positive emotions; build mastery; cope ahead; Please—treat physical illness; balance eating; avoid mood-altering substances; maintain good sleep; get exercise
> **DEAR MAN:** describe, express, assert, reinforce, mindful, appear, negotiate
> **GIVE:** gentle; interested; validate; easy manner
> **"WHAT" skills** help to become mindful by focusing on the present moment, including thoughts, physical sensations, and emotions
> **"HOW" skills** help to learn how to be both mindful and nonjudgmental in daily life.

Table 9.1 DBT and yin yoga

DBT module	Skills acquired	Practices that can be utilized in yoga	Yin poses
Distress tolerance	Distraction Self-soothing	REST Radical acceptance Using the senses	Wide-Knee Child Tadpole Frog
Mindfulness	Nonjudgmental awareness of thoughts, emotions, physical sensations, and actions	Wise Mind WHAT skills HOW skills	Butterfly Supported Bridge Legs Up the Wall pose
Emotion regulation	Reduce emotional suffering	ABC PLEASE Opposite action to change emotions	Select personal "easy" yin pose Select "challenging" yin pose
Interpersonal effectiveness	Healthy assertion of needs and reducing conflict	DEAR MAN GIVE	Relaxation (with guided meditation) Seated meditation (spoken aloud with partner)

INTERNAL FAMILY SYSTEMS: WORKING WITH OUR DIFFERENT PERSONALITY PARTS

I was introduced to Internal Family Systems in 2007, about a decade into my career as a psychologist. I was struck by how this model—which emphasizes "parts" or different inner voices or subpersonalities inside of us—can provide a helpful and compassionate pathway to working with negative thoughts, emotions, and behaviors, and the ever-present inner critic. Created by marriage and family therapist Richard Schwartz in the 1990s, IFS has become a well-recognized model for treating a variety of long-standing psychological conditions, including depression, anxiety, trauma, eating disorders, and relationship difficulties. According to Schwartz:

> It is the nature of the human mind to be subdivided into an indeterminate number of subpersonalities called parts (most clients identify and work with between 5 and 15 parts through the course of therapy). These parts are conceptualized as inner people of different ages, temperaments, talents, desires, who together form an internal family or tribe. This internal family organizes itself in the same way as other human systems and reflects the organization of the systems around it.[15]

What I particularly appreciate about this model is how Schwartz emphasizes the value in *all* parts. Instead of trying to get one especially troublesome part of ourselves (or the message from that part) to go away, this model teaches how to engage with each of our parts, to explore what they need, how they feel, and what important messages they have for us from their experiences. IFS also addresses this idea of a Self (with a capital S). Schwartz elaborates that:

> Everyone has a seat of consciousness at their core, which we call the Self. From birth this Self has all of the necessary qualities of good leadership, such as compassion, perspective, curiosity, acceptance, and confidence. It does not have to develop through stages. As a result, the Self makes the best inner leader and will engender balance and harmony inside if parts allow it to lead.[16]

However, for many of us, especially if we have experienced trauma or deep wounding as children, these parts may blend their feelings, experiences, and pain with the Self, which can interfere with the Self's ability to lead a life that is meaningful, purposeful, and joyful. If there is a safe environment (through a therapist as an expert guide), we can reorganize our system by working with our parts through active engagement with them and learn how to restore harmony and Self leadership.

Given that many people have experienced childhood wounds and sometimes traumatic events, the work of IFS must be done carefully and safely with a trained therapist so as not to overwhelm or re-traumatize the client before sufficiently establishing the Self's ability to witness, listen, and empathize, and help these parts to live in the present with their fears sufficiently comforted and their burdens of the past released.

In yin yoga, I utilize IFS in a very careful and specific context to ensure each client's safety and stability: rather than focusing directly on the subpersonality parts which can create stress, I focus instead on strengthening Self leadership. By working on the core qualities of the Self (what Schwartz calls the 8 C's), *curiosity, calm, confidence, connectedness, clarity, creativity, courage, and compassion,* students can begin to feel the power of having more capacity to be with all of their experiences (feelings, sensations, inner critic, voices—their *parts*).[17]

As with DBT, these IFS techniques should only be utilized by a trained mental health professional with specific training in IFS and should include supervision by an IFS-trained instructor. In Table 9.2 I describe the Self qualities that can be explored in yin poses, utilizing inquiry questions that allow students to practice mobilizing these strengths.

Table 9.2 IFS and yin yoga practice

Self-quality	Inquiry prompt	Yin pose
Calmness	What would create a sense of calmness and ease in this moment?	Seated meditation Supported Bridge/Fish
Clarity	Using all of your senses, what is happening in this moment?	Body Scan meditation iRest yoga *nidra*
Curiosity	Explore a new edge in this pose by increasing or decreasing the intensity	Sphinx/Seal Figure Four
Compassion	Place your hand on your heart and use one of the following phrases, or select one of your own: "I can be this" "I am willing to stay" "This is hard"	Butterfly
Confidence	Recognize personal sense of grace by selecting one of the following phrases: "I am loved" "I am love" "I am whole" "I am healthy" "I feel my basic goodness"	Saddle or Supported Bridge
Courage	"I am strong" "Even though this is____[hard/ uncomfortable/upsetting], I can stay here"	Frog or Wide-Knee Child pose
Creativity	"I am in the flow" "I feel my aliveness" "I am at home in my body"	Start in Dangle (Standing Forward Fold) 90–120 seconds Move into squat or supported squat using block 90–120 seconds
Connectedness	Sense your connection with those around you, in the room, outside the room, your family, friends, colleagues. Imagine sending them wishes of care and love (lovingkindness phrases) Sense your connection with a favorite spot in nature	Legs Up the Wall/Chair

ENDNOTES

1   Hofmann, A.A., Hofmann, S.G., Asnaani, A., Vonk, I.J., *et al.* (2012) 'The efficacy of cognitive behavioral therapy: A review of meta-analyses.' *Cognitive Therapy Research, 36,* 5, 427–440.

2   Gaudiano, B. (2008) 'Cognitive-behavioral therapies: Achievements and challenges.' *Evidence-Based Mental Health, 11,* 1, 5–7.

3   Gaudiano, B. (2008) 'Cognitive-behavioral therapies: Achievements and challenges.' *Evidence-Based Mental Health, 11,* 1, 5–7.

4   Hofmann, A.A., *et al.* (2012) 'The efficacy of cognitive behavioral therapy: A review of meta-analyses.' *Cognitive Therapy Research, 36,* 5, 427–440.

5   Gaudiano, B. (2008) 'Cognitive-behavioral therapies: Achievements and challenges.' *Evidence-Based Mental Health, 11,* 1, 5–7.

6   Amen, D. (1998) *Change Your Brain, Change Your Life.* New York: Random House, p.56.

7   Amen, D. (1998) *Change Your Brain, Change Your Life.* New York: Random House, p.63.

8   Linehan, M.M. (1993) *Cognitive-Behavioral Treatment of Borderline Personality Disorder.* New York: Guilford Press.

9   DiGiorgio, K., Glass, C., and Arnkoff, D. (2010) 'Therapists' use of DBT: A survey study of clinical practice.' *Cognitive and Behavioral Practice, 17,* 2, 213–221.

10 Dimeff, L., and Linehan, M. (2001) 'Dialectical behavior therapy in a nutshell.' *California Psychologist, 34,* 10–13.

11 Dimeff, L., and Linehan, M. (2001) 'Dialectical behavior therapy in a nutshell.' *California Psychologist, 34,* 10–13.

12 Linehan, M.M. (1993) *Cognitive-Behavioral Treatment of Borderline Personality Disorder.* New York: Guilford Press.

13 McKay, M., Wood, J.C., and Brantley, J. (2010) *The Dialectical Behavior Therapy Skills Workbook: Practical DBT exercises for learning mindfulness, interpersonal effectiveness, emotion regulation and distress tolerance.* Oakland, CA: New Harbinger.

14 DiGiorgio, K., Glass, C., and Arnkoff, D. (2010) 'Therapists' use of DBT: A survey study of clinical practice.' *Cognitive and Behavioral Practice, 17,* 2, 213–221.

15 Schwartz, R., and Sweezy, M. (2020) *Internal Family Systems Therapy* (2nd ed.). New York: The Guilford Press, p.39.

16 Schwartz, R., and Sweezy, M. (2020) *Internal Family Systems Therapy* (2nd ed.). New York: The Guilford Press, p.38.

17 Schwartz, R., and Sweezy, M. (2020) *Internal Family Systems Therapy* (2nd ed.). New York: The Guilford Press, p 45.

— Chapter 10 —

YIN YOGA FOR
DEPRESSION

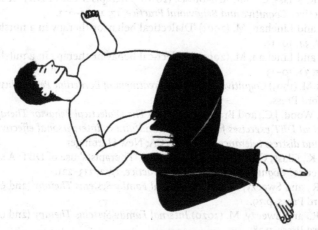

Twists can help gently release physical and emotional tension, making room for healing

One day, my client Penny did not show up for her weekly yoga therapy session. Concerned, I called her, and she answered the phone in a barely audible voice. I asked her if she was okay and she said, "I feel so depressed...I can't even bring myself to get out of bed and take a shower, never mind come in to see you." She had already reached out to her psychiatrist, who was considering a medication increase. Over the next few minutes on the phone, I asked her if she could imagine even the most basic self-care plan for the day. I pointed out that due to her depression, her energy was so low she was like a car engine "running on empty." Therefore, even small tasks seemed insurmountable.

To "conserve her energy," I invited her to do a few short practices together with me while she was in bed if she was willing. She quietly said that she would try. I began by leading a simple three-part breath *pranayama* practice to gently and gradually expand her breath cycle and particularly focus on lengthening the in-breath. We did this for five breath cycles. I checked in again and asked her if she was willing to continue. She agreed to continue so I led her through alternate nostril breathing, emphasizing the three components of the practice: *inhale* through one nostril and hold, *exhale* through the other nostril, and *inhale* through the same nostril and continue. We did this for about two minutes. I checked in again and asked her how she was feeling. Her voice was still quiet, but she sounded more alert. "Okay," she said tentatively. I asked her if she would be willing to do a couple of gentle yoga poses while she rested in bed. She agreed and we went through a few gentle stretches, including Banana-asana (reclining side bend), Twist (reclining), and Knees in the Chest. When we concluded this short five-minute practice, her voice was louder and clearer. "I am going to get up now. That actually felt pretty good." I invited her to stay in bed for a minute longer and led her through a visualization where she imagined how she wanted to use her energy in a way that would bring soothing and ease to her day. She agreed to conserve her energy so that she could slowly build up some more resources over the next few days and rescheduled her appointment for later in the week.

When Penny came into her session, she looked tired and drawn. However, her voice was strong, and her eyes looked alert and bright. She said that she "barely got through the last three days" but continued to practice the breathing exercises a few times a day and that they seemed to help. I asked her if she would be willing to do a few standing breath exercises before we sat for our session. She agreed and we began some simple Sun Breaths, spending about ten breaths in Forward Fold before slowly inhaling back up to standing. She reported that she felt some heat and energy in her body. She sat down in the chair across from me and stated that she felt ready to "work."

Penny's depression responded to a slow titration up of breath work and gentle movement instead of trying to override her nervous system. She responded to this slow build-up and was able to utilize more of her natural coping skills once she felt more energy flow in her system. If I had tried to get her to go for a walk or do a more strenuous Vinyasa practice, I would have likely met a lot of resistance as she simply did not have enough energy (mental/physical/emotional) to meet those task demands. Working with clients who experience depression requires a careful assessment of energy level, window of tolerance, and motivation to stay with a practice. Penny enjoyed feeling the slow improvement in her energy level which allowed her to combat her lethargy.

DEPRESSION

Depression is one of the most common mental health disorders around the world. According to the World Health Organization, more than 264 million people of all ages experience depression.[1] The estimated lifetime prevalence is 10 percent of the general population and may be as high as 20 percent in clinical populations including outpatient and inpatient psychiatric facilities.[2] While many of us experience day-to-day fluctuations in our mood that may cause us to feel sad or down, depression can be a significant and serious health condition. Major depressive disorder (MDD), in particular, can result in significant and sometimes severe impairment in a person's ability to carry out daily activities. It is the most common mood disorder in the United States, with a lifetime prevalence estimated at 14.4 percent.[3]

According to the World Health Organization, when a person experiences a depressed mood (or loss of pleasure in activities) nearly every day for at least two weeks, it is considered a depressive episode. In addition, they may experience other symptoms, including poor concentration, feelings of guilt, low self-esteem, hopelessness about the future, suicidal thoughts, and changes in sleep, appetite, weight, and energy. The severity of the symptoms (mild, moderate, or severe) depends on the number of the symptoms as well the impact of these symptoms on a person's daily functioning. Mood disorders range from a single event to recurrent events (at least two depressive episodes). The National Institute of Mental Health (NIMH) describes different forms of depression, including *persistent depressive disorder* or dysthymia, where an individual experiences a depressed mood for at least two years; *premenstrual dysphoric disorder (PMDD)*, which includes depression and other mood-related symptoms prior to the start of a woman's period; *postpartum depression* (feelings of extreme sadness, anxiety, fatigue) which can occur for women after delivery of a baby and interferes with caring for their babies or themselves; psychotic depression, which includes a combination of both depressed mood and psychotic symptoms such as delusions or hallucinations; *seasonal affective disorder*, which typically occurs in the winter months and returns every year; and *bipolar disorder*, which includes both major depressive episodes and manic or irritable moods.[4]

Examples of these disorders, additional types of depression, and specific diagnostic criteria can be found in the fifth edition of the *Diagnostic and Statistical Manual* (DSM-5).[5]

In the United States, an estimated 17.3 million adults have experienced at least one major depressive episode, with the highest prevalence found in young adults aged 18–25.[6] (See Figure 10.1 for prevalence breakdown by sex, age, and race.) In terms of severity, of the adults who have experienced an episode of major depression, 64 percent had "severe impairment" compared to 36 percent "without severe impairment." Severe impairment can be debilitating in terms of inability to work or maintain roles and responsibilities, and possible hospitalization. Major depressive disorder is considered a chronic condition in that most individuals suffering from it are likely to have recurrent episodes.[7] In addition to the debilitating symptoms, major depression contributes to mortality. According to the Centers for Disease Control and Prevention, suicide was the tenth leading cause of death in 2018, with over 48,000 people dying each year.[8] It is estimated that at least a third of these deaths are accounted for by those experiencing major depression.[9]

Bipolar disorder is another type of mood disorder, which includes episodes of intense emotional states that can last days to weeks. These mood episodes are classified as manic or hypomanic/depressive in nature. There are three different types of bipolar disorders: bipolar I, bipolar II, and cyclothymic disorder. Bipolar I is diagnosed when an individual who has also experienced at least one major depressive episode lasting two weeks or more experiences at least one manic episode—characterized by an extreme increase in energy and leading to significant disruption in daily life—that lasts at least one week. Bipolar II is diagnosed if an individual experiences at least one hypomanic episode—characterized by less severe manic symptoms that last four days or more and do not lead to a major disruption in functioning—and one major depressive episode lasting at least two weeks. Finally, the mildest form of bipolar disorder is cyclothymic disorder, which involves more mood swings that occur frequently with hypomanic and depressive symptoms for a period of at least two years, but with less severe intensity than major depressive episodes or mania.

For the purposes of this chapter, I will focus primarily on major depression, as it represents the most common mood disorder that many clinicians and yoga therapists will encounter in their work. Most of the practices and recommendations in this chapter are applicable to the other mood disorders described above, but as always, it is important to consider the individual rather than just the diagnosis when developing effective practices to ease suffering.

Mental health clinicians and researchers have long been exploring the key factors for depression, and largely have come to believe that there is an interplay between stress, the environment, and an individual's genetics, including neurochemistry. Life stressors, particularly if they create a sense of "learned helplessness" where people no longer feel that they can control a situation, lead to a higher risk of depression.[10] Stressors that occur during childhood and are more extreme, known as "adverse childhood experiences," have also been shown to increase an individual's risk of depression.[11]

With major depressive disorder, there is a more chronic cycle of depression suggesting what researchers call a "kindling" effect, in which each episode (especially those that are prolonged or untreated) increases the likelihood of another recurrence. This can create an ongoing cycle of MDD that might have started with a life stressor that caused an initial depression; then, over time, the depression causes additional life stressors in many important social and daily living spheres. This can eventually create what researchers call "allostatic overload," when an individual can become permanently disabled because they simply do not have the coping skills to manage the levels of stress they are enduring.[12]

Treatment for major depression is vital to help people regain central aspects of their lives, but over one-third of those diagnosed do not receive treatment. Those who do receive treatment typically receive a combination of professional therapy sessions and medication.[13] (See Figure 10.2 for types of treatment received for Major Depressive Episode.) Barriers to treatment are primarily cost-related, but also include a lack of knowledge about where to go for treatment, and fear of being committed or forced to take medications.[14]

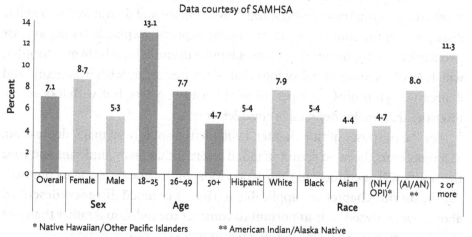

* Native Hawaiian/Other Pacific Islanders   ** American Indian/Alaska Native

Figure 10.1 Past-year prevalence of major depressive episodes among US adults (2017)[15]

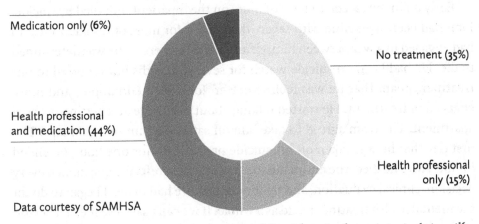

Medication only (6%)

No treatment (35%)

Health professional
and medication (44%)

Health professional
only (15%)

Data courtesy of SAMHSA

Figure 10.2 Past-year treatment received among adults with major depressive episode (2017)[16]

As a psychologist and yoga therapist, I encounter many clients who are experiencing the full range of different types of depression, from mild adjustment disorders to severe MDD with suicidal ideation. Most of my clients have already had long treatment histories prior to seeing me, including the use of antidepressant medications, psychotherapy, and sometimes more invasive procedures, including electroconvulsive therapy (ECT) and transmagnetic stimulation (TMS), with varying degrees of symptom relief. According to the research, the most effective treatment for depression is antidepressant medication, followed closely by cognitive behavioral therapy.[17] However, the research also shows that despite the expanding number of medications and other types of psychiatric therapies, nearly half of those experiencing MDD do not respond adequately to these treatments to achieve true remission.[18, 19]

When I worked in inpatient psychiatric units, I would often meet clients who felt hopeless and let down by the mental health system. They would report that they felt like they were treated like laboratory rats when they were put on the newest types of medications, or that their reports of side-effects such as weight gain and loss of sex drive, which created even more emotional distress, were often minimized, or ignored.

As part of that same mental health system, I would feel both distress and helplessness when I encountered these clients. I would often go through the motions of encouraging them not to give up, to keep trying new medications, to go to their therapy groups, while at the same time I observed the pervasiveness of their loss of interest or their growing sense of hopelessness. It is devastating for clinicians when a client dies of suicide. The feeling of loss, self-blame, and grief often causes us to question the very purpose of our work and erodes our deepest convictions about the power of psychotherapy to heal.

Early on in my career, a client of mine on the inpatient unit died by suicide. John had been struggling with severe depression for most of his adult life and had engaged in a war between himself and his caregivers, as he was determined to die. He had been on suicide watch for several months but reported to our treatment team that he was feeling better. John seemed happier and more engaged in treatment. He started talking about discharge and getting his own apartment. The team agreed to take him off safety precautions gradually. The first day that he was taken off his suicide precautions for one hour, he ended his life. After he died, the entire inpatient unit was bereft. We questioned every decision, clinical evaluation, and treatment plan we had made. I began to doubt the mental health treatment field as a whole. If we can't save the life of a person who is obviously crying out for help, what is it that we are really doing? Over the next weeks and months, the hospital did its review, its "critical incident rounds," and came up with new safety recommendations to make it more difficult for clients to hurt themselves within the hospital environment.

The hospital moved on to other issues and that suicide became part of the past. But I felt haunted. I thought, there must be other ways to help people heal from depression that we are not accessing. It was at that time that I began my own meditation and yoga practice to address my own struggles with anxiety. Somewhere deep in the back of my mind, I started to wonder if these same practices might support even my most depressed clients.

Over the next decade or more, I witnessed the power of yin yoga practice for clients with depression. It can be a lifeline as clients begin to feel some connection returning with their bodies, and begin to find a gentler space to inhabit, at least when they are on the yoga mat. In addition, the fact of being in a yoga community with other people who are also trying to find their way can provide the necessary connection to reduce feelings of isolation and separateness.

RESEARCH ON YOGA FOR DEPRESSION

Many individuals seek mind-body or complementary therapies, including yoga, for depression and other mental health conditions, because traditional treatments may be inadequate or ineffective in managing their symptoms—especially for those suffering from episodic depression, in which the symptoms recur over months and even years without full remission.[20, 21] Research over the past two decades has indicated that yoga can have a beneficial impact on MDD and other mood disorders.[22] Studies have shown that yoga can decrease depression severity,[23, 24] increase awareness of feelings and bodily sensations,[25] minimize rumination,[26] increase a sense of calm and well-being,[27, 28, 29] increase self-compassion,[30, 31, 32] and improve mental focus.[33] Systematic reviews of different yoga studies have concluded that yoga interventions, primarily Hatha yoga (which has been most widely studied), have been effective in reducing depression. However, these reviews also noted methodological limitations in these studies in that there were small sample sizes, lack of longitudinal studies, and heterogeneity of randomized control trials.[34, 35]

In addition to exploring the effectiveness of yoga for depression, researchers have also begun to hypothesize about the underlying mechanisms that create these positive effects on mood and overall well-being. Some preliminary studies suggest that yoga practice can increase neurotransmitter production and release neurochemicals thought to play a major role in depression, specifically dopamine,[36, 37] serotonin,[38] and gamma-aminobutyric acid (GABA).[39, 40]

Other hypotheses for the mechanisms of yoga for depression involve the stress hormone cortisol. While the studies around cortisol levels and yoga are quite limited, with challenges in consistency and methodology, researchers continue to explore how decreasing cortisol may be integral to how yoga decreases depression, based on studies with breast cancer survivors and those suffering from alcohol dependence.[41, 42, 43, 44] Other studies have looked at how yoga might impact specific circuits in the brain in terms of changes of blood flow and cellular metabolism, particularly in the areas of the prefrontal cortex that can improve stress control and self-regulation and are key to managing depression.[45]

It is important to note that many of these studies are preliminary or are hypothetical in terms of the mechanisms of how yoga might decrease depression. Furthermore, I want to be clear that I do not believe that yoga alone is sufficient to treat serious forms of depression, given the complexity of its causes and its often chronic nature. However, I do strongly believe that yoga can be an important complementary or supportive part of a holistic treatment approach to depression, which may also include medication, psychotherapy, and psychoeducation. When I began to integrate yin yoga into my work with clients who suffered from depression, I discovered new pathways to help them manage stress and improve their overall quality of life.

YIN YOGA FOR DEPRESSION

When I first started introducing traditional Hatha yoga practices to my clients in the psychiatric hospital, I found that some of them immediately benefited from the movement, flow, and strengthening aspects of the practice. However, many of my clients, particularly those that were struggling with major depression or other mood disorders, shied away from yoga practice altogether. When I asked whether they would be interested in participating, I would hear similar themes in their responses: "I'm too tired," "I don't have the energy," "I don't feel up to it." In trying to find a doorway into introducing them to yoga, I suggested that we would just do a few poses and they would not even have to get off the floor; I would offer a maximum of two or three poses followed by a guided meditation. Interestingly, they seemed to be more energized after the practice, even though the poses were largely static and not particularly challenging.

I began starting off most of my therapeutic classes this way, with static poses and longer holdings so that I would not immediately overwhelm those clients who were depressed and had low energy. After my yin training, I utilized this same idea of starting with a set of two to three poses at relatively low levels of sensation for my clients who were depressed. I invited them to stay with sensations in the lower range of one to two on the yin sensation scale and provided them with a gentle inquiry to notice their experience of being connected to their bodies. I found that some poses in combination were particularly potent in terms of shifting energy from sadness to more ease and lightness, using TCM-influenced energetic sequences including ones that target the Heart/Lung/Small Intestine organ/meridian pairs. These included heart-opening poses such as Reclining Butterfly, Supported Fish, Quarter Dog variations, and different laterals and twists, including Wide-Knee Child with Twist and Reclining Twists.

Sarah Powers describes how when Heart *Qi* is out of balance, "there may be a propensity for acute sadness, desperation, joylessness, depression, and estrangement when depleted."[46] I find that encouraging my clients to take a few of these shapes brings them more balance, both emotionally and energetically. Powers goes on to say, "when heart chi is healthy, we feel warm, nourished, and nourishing, able to contact innate joy, inner peace, and harmony, and able to build healthy relationships."[47]

Although it felt counterintuitive to use slow static poses with gentle stimulation as opposed to rhythmic muscular engagement to increase a sense of vitality, I was amazed how many clients reported that they felt better several hours after a class. Their nervous system, sometimes stuck for days, weeks, months, or even years, in this hypoaroused state, began to transform with these gentle, energy-shifting poses. I found that maintaining a three-times-per-week schedule in the morning that ended with a guided relaxation practice (yoga *nidra* or body scan) produced shifts in mood, energy level, and even the type of self-talk, favoring more compassionate and less self-recriminating speech. It was beneficial for my clients to largely stick with the same basic poses, and I invited only small incremental changes in terms of level of sensation and duration of holding the pose.

Depression is one of the most common conditions that I come across in my clinical work as a psychologist. Many of my clients have tried multiple interventions to manage their depression with varying degrees of success in decreasing their symptoms and few maintaining full remission from depression. I have found that integrating yin yoga and mindfulness practices into daily life for those struggling with depression can play an important role in symptom reduction, improved quality of life, and overall mood stability. I have been amazed to see some of my clients remain in full remission from what was once a debilitating mood disorder by committing to a daily yoga and meditation practice along with ongoing psychiatric care.

ENDNOTES

1   www.who.int/news-room/fact-sheets/detail/depression
2   Tolentino, J.C., and Schmidt, S.L. (2018) 'DSM-5 criteria and depression severity: Implications for clinical practice.' *Frontiers in Psychiatry, 9,* 450.
3   Kessler, R.C., Petukhova, M., Sampson, N.A., Zaslavsky, A.M., and Wittchen, H.U. (2012) 'Twelve-month and lifetime prevalence and lifetime morbid risk of anxiety and mood disorders in the United States.' *International Journal of Methods in Psychiatric Research, 21,* 169–184.
4   www.nimh.nih.gov/health/topics/depression
5   American Psychiatric Association (2013) *Diagnostic and Statistical Manual of Mental Disorders* (5th ed.) (DSM-5). Arlington, VA: APA.
6   Amat, J., Paul, E., Zarza, C., Watkins, L., and Maier, S. (2006) 'Previous experience with behavioral control over stress blocks the behavioral and dorsal raphe nucleus activating effects of later uncontrollable stress: Role of ventral medial prefrontal cortex.' *Journal of Neuroscience, 26,* 51, 13264–13272.
7   Maletic, V., Robinson, M., Oakes, T., Iyengar, S., Ball, S.G., and Russell, J. (2007) 'Neurobiology of depression: An integrated view of key findings.' *International Journal of Clinical Practice, 61,* 12, 2030–2040.
8   www.nimh.nih.gov/health/statistics/major-depression.shtml
9   www.nimh.nih.gov/health/statistics/major-depression.shtml
10 Amat, J., Paul, E., Zarza, C., Watkins, L., and Maier, S. (2006) 'Previous experience with behavioral control over stress blocks the behavioral and dorsal raphe nucleus activating effects of later uncontrollable stress: Role of ventral medial prefrontal cortex.' *Journal of Neuroscience, 26,* 51, 13264–13272.
11 Maletic, V., Robinson, M., Oakes, T., Iyengar, S., Ball, S.G., and Russell, J. (2007) 'Neurobiology of depression: An integrated view of key findings.' *International Journal of Clinical Practice, 61,* 12, 2030–2040.
12 Kinser, P., Goehler, L., and Taylor, A.G. (2012) 'How might yoga help depression? A neurobiological perspective.' *Explore, 8,* 2, 118–126.

13 Maletic, V., Robinson, M., Oakes, T., Iyengar, S., Ball, S.G., and Russell, J. (2007) 'Neurobiology of depression: An integrated view of key findings.' *International Journal of Clinical Practice, 61, 12,* 2030–2040.

14 Chekroud, A., Foster, D., Zheutlin, A.B., Gerhard, D.M., *et al.* (2018) 'Predicting barriers to treatment for depression in a US national sample: A cross-sectional, proof-of-concept study.' *Psychiatric Services, 69,* 8, 927–934.

15 www.nimh.nih.gov/health/statistics/major-depression.shtml

16 www.nimh.nih.gov/health/statistics/major-depression.shtml

17 Hillhouse, T.M., and Porter, J.H. (2015) 'A brief history of the development of antidepressant drugs: From monoamines to glutamate.' *Experimental and Clinical Psychopharmacology, 23,* 1, 1–21.

18 Hillhouse, T.M., and Porter, J.H. (2015) 'A brief history of the development of antidepressant drugs: From monoamines to glutamate.' *Experimental and Clinical Psychopharmacology, 23,* 1, 1–21.

19 Fava, M., and Davidson, K.G. (1996) 'Definition and epidemiology of treatment-resistant depression.' *Psychiatric Clinics of North America, 19,* 179–200.

20 Boschloo, L., Bekhuis, E., Weitz, E.S., Reijnders, M., *et al.* (2019) 'The symptom-specific efficacy of antidepressant medication vs. cognitive behavioral therapy in the treatment of depression: Results from an individual client data meta-analysis.' *World Psychiatry, 18,* 2, 183–191.

21 Fava, M., and Davidson, K.G. (1996) 'Definition and epidemiology of treatment-resistant depression.' *Psychiatric Clinics of North America, 19,* 179–200.

22 Cramer, H., Lauche, R., Langhorst, J., and Dobos, G. (2013) 'Yoga for depression: A systematic review and meta-analysis.' *Depression and Anxiety, 00,* 1–16.

23 Cramer, H., Lauche, R., Langhorst, J., and Dobos, G. (2013) 'Yoga for depression: A systematic review and meta-analysis.' *Depression and Anxiety, 00,* 1–16.

24 Bridges, L., and Sharma, M. (2017) 'The efficacy of yoga as a form of treatment for depression.' *Journal of Evidence-Based Complementary & Alternative Medicine, 22,* 4, 1017–1028.

25 Meyer, H.B., Katsman, A., Sones, A.C., *et al.* (2012) 'Yoga as an ancillary treatment for neurological and psychiatric disorders: A review.' *Journal of Neuropsychiatry and Clinical Neuroscience, 24,* 152–164.

26 Schuver, K., and Lewis, B. (2016) 'Mindfulness-based yoga intervention for women with depression.' *Complementary Therapies in Medicine, 26,* 85–91.

27 Kinser, P., Goehler, L., and Taylor, A.G. (2012) 'How might yoga help depression? A neurobiological perspective.' *Explore, 8,* 2, 118–126.

28 Brown, R.P., and Gerbarg, P.L. (2005) 'Sudarshan Kriya Yogic breathing in the treatment of stress, anxiety, and depression: Part I—Neurophysiological model.' *Journal of Complementary and Alternative Medicine, 11,* 4, 189–201.

29 Brown, R.P., and Gerbarg, P.L. (2005) 'Sudarshan Kriya Yogic breathing in the treatment of stress, anxiety, and depression: Part II—Clinical applications and guidelines.' *Journal of Complementary and Alternative Medicine, 11,* 4, 711–717.

30 Jonsson, G., Franzen, L., Nystrom, M., and Davis, P. (2020) 'Integrating yoga with psychological group-treatment for mixed depression and anxiety in primary healthcare: An exploratory pilot study.' *Complementary Therapies in Clinical Practice, 41,* 101250.

31 Gard, T., Brach, N., Holzer, B., Noggle, J., Conboy, L., and Lazar, S. (2012) 'Effects of a yoga-based intervention for young adults on quality of life and perceived stress: The potential mediating roles of mindfulness and self-compassion.' *Journal of Positive Psychology, 7,* 3, 165–175.

32 Snaith, N., Schultz, T., Proeve, M., and Rasmussen, P. (2018) 'Mindfulness, self-compassion, anxiety and depression measures in South Australian yoga participants: Implications for designing a yoga intervention.' *Complementary Therapies in Clinical Practice, 32,* 92–99.

33 Meyer, H.B., Katsman, A., Sones, A.C., *et al.* (2012) 'Yoga as an ancillary treatment for neurological and psychiatric disorders: A review.' *Journal of Neuropsychiatry and Clinical Neuroscience, 24,* 152–164.

34 Cramer, H., Lauche, R., Langhorst, J., and Dobos, G. (2013) 'Yoga for depression: A systematic review and meta-analysis.' *Depression and Anxiety, 00,* 1–16.

35 Bridges, L., and Sharma, M. (2017) 'The efficacy of yoga as a form of treatment for depression.' *Journal of Evidence-Based Complementary & Alternative Medicine, 22,* 4, 1017–1028.

36 Kjaer, T.W., Bertelsen, C., Piccini, P., *et al.* (2002) 'Increased dopamine tone during meditation-induced change of consciousness.' *Brain Research. Cognitive Brain Research, 13,* 255–259.

37 Kinser, P., Goehler, L., and Taylor, A.G. (2012) 'How might yoga help depression? A neurobiological perspective.' *Explore, 8,* 2, 118–126.

38 Kinser, P., Goehler, L., and Taylor, A.G. (2012) 'How might yoga help depression? A neurobiological perspective.' *Explore, 8,* 2, 118–126.

39 Streeter, C.C., Gerbarg, P.L., Saper, R.B., *et al.* (2012) 'Effects of yoga on the autonomic nervous system, gamma-aminobutyric-acid, and allostasis in epilepsy, depression, and post-traumatic stress disorder.' *Medical Hypotheses, 78,* 571–579.

40 Streeter, C.C., Whitfield, T.H., Owen, L., *et al.* (2010) 'Effects of yoga versus walking on mood, anxiety, and brain GABA levels: A randomized controlled MRS study.' *Journal of Alternative and Complementary Medicine, 16,* 11, 1145–1152.

41 Chong, C.S., Tsunaka, M., Tsang, H.W., *et al.* (2011) 'Effects of yoga on stress management in healthy adults: A systematic review.' *Alternative Therapies in Health and Medicine, 17,* 32–38.

42 Vedamurthachar, A., Janakiramaiah, N., Hegde, J.M., *et al.* (2006) 'Antidepressant efficacy and hormonal effects of Sudarshana Kriya Yoga (SKY) in alcohol dependent individuals.' *Journal of Affective Disorders, 94,* 249–253.

43 Vadiraja, H.S., Raghavendra, R.M., Nagarathna, R., *et al.* (2009) 'Effects of a yoga program on cortisol rhythm and mood states in early breast cancer clients undergoing adjuvant radiotherapy: A randomized controlled trial.' *Integrative Cancer Therapies, 8,* 37–46.

44 Banasik, J., Williams, H., Haberman, M., *et al.* (2011) 'Effect of Iyengar yoga practice on fatigue and diurnal salivary cortisol concentration in breast cancer survivors.' *Journal of the American Academy of Nurse Practitioners, 23,* 135–142.

45 Kinser, P., Goehler, L., and Taylor, A.G. (2012) 'How might yoga help depression? A neurobiological perspective.' *Explore, 8,* 2, 118–126.

46 Powers, S. (2008) *Insight Yoga.* Boulder, CO: Shambhala Publications, p.88.

47 Powers, S. (2008) *Insight Yoga.* Boulder, CO: Shambhala Publications, p.88.

— Chapter 11 —

YIN YOGA FOR ANXIETY

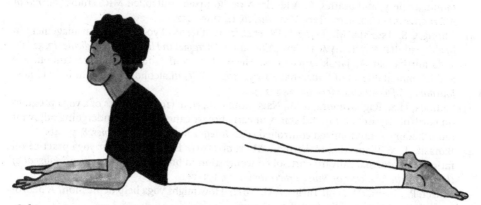

Sphinx pose provides a low intensity backbend that can reduce nervous system over-reactivity

The first time I spoke with Cassie on the phone as she shared that she wanted to do some yoga with me, I was struck by the slightly pressured, almost panicky sound in her voice. "I am really struggling right now," she said. "I keep thinking that I am going to pass out."

Cassie had a history of unexplained fainting episodes that would occur at the most inopportune times, including when she was at a meeting with her boss, at a rehearsal dinner for her wedding, and at a recent work picnic. She was a healthy 25-year-old woman with an otherwise unremarkable medical history. She had seen multiple specialists, including a neurologist, a cardiologist, and an endocrinologist, but they could not find anything wrong. Ultimately, they settled on a diagnosis of vasovagal syncope, a relatively common and not life-threatening condition that occurs when the body over-reacts to certain triggers. Even though it was not a serious medical condition, Cassie was becoming increasingly anxious about the thought of having another fainting episode and described how humiliated she felt when she fainted in front of a large group of people.

When I met Cassie for our first session, she was friendly, bubbly, and spoke rapidly about her upcoming wedding, job opportunity, and graduate school dissertation. She was clearly a motivated and hard-working woman with a positive future to look forward to. I was curious if she was able to slow down and do a few body-based practices. I led her through some basic breath awareness exercises. She closed her eyes tightly and I watched her wring her hands while she sat silently without any other perceptible movement. After a few minutes, I asked her what she was observing.

Her eyes flew open, and she said, "I could not focus at all. All I kept thinking about was what I need to do next today." I asked her to rate her anxiety on a scale of one to ten and she stated it was at an eight. Clearly, Cassie was not going to settle easily with meditation or grounding practices just then. I invited her to stand up with me and begin to shake out her body, beginning with the arms and legs. I began to speed up the shaking and asked her to follow my lead. I added hips, head, and shoulders to the arms and legs, and we continued to shake our whole bodies for another minute or so. We were both breathing more heavily, and I saw how her eyes—which had looked alarmed after the first grounding meditation—began to soften, and she said, a bit breathless, "Wow, I was literally shaking off my stress."

From there, we began a series of gentle yoga movements, including Half Sun Salutations, Dancing Warriors, and Goddess/Five-Pointed Star. I asked her if we could try to slow down for a few moments but still maintain a sense of flow and movement. I invited her to take a Forward Fold and begin by swaying back and forth and then come into relative stillness. I asked her to focus on her breath and the sensations of the body. I watched how her back softened and her breathing slowed down.

After about 90 seconds, I invited her to squat. Once again, I asked her if she was able to focus on the sensations in her legs, back, and whole body along with her breath. I saw that her eyes remained alert but were now soft, as she remained in the squat for 90 seconds. I invited her to come down onto the floor and take a seated Caterpillar with the same focus on the body and breath. She stayed in the pose for two minutes and I asked her if she could stay for five more breaths. She nodded and I saw her shoulders soften and her breath deepen. I invited her to sit up and take a cross-legged position. With her eyes open, I asked her once more to come into mindfulness of her breath. This time, her body was alert but relaxed. Her breath was slow and even. Her eyes remained open but slightly out of focus. After three minutes, I asked her to rate her anxiety. She stated she was at a two.

"Wow, I don't know what just happened, but I like it!" she said happily.

Cassie was able to respond to a yin and meditation practice only after she had moved some of the tension and anxiety that was coursing through her like a waterfall. Through the shaking movement, she was able to become more and more present to her experience. By the time she took yin shapes, she was able to stay connected to her body and her breath for longer periods of time. Her initial response to the opening meditation signaled to me that her nervous system would not tolerate a "traditional" yin practice right away. But placed at the end of a movement practice, the yin poses allowed her to feel deeply soothed and much more at ease.

ANXIETY STATISTICS

Anxiety is the number one mental health issue worldwide, with an estimated 275 million people suffering from some type of anxiety disorder (about 4% of the global population).[1] It is also the most prevalent psychiatric disorder in the United States. Statistics range from 18 to 20 percent of adults experiencing some type of anxiety disorder per year, with higher incidence among females (23%) than males (14%). (See Figure 11.1 for prevalence breakdown by gender and age.) Even more striking is that an estimated 30 percent of US adults have experienced anxiety at some point during their lifetimes.[2]

Anxiety disorders often begin during childhood and adolescence. Like depression, the severity of impairment due to anxiety can range from mild (43%) through moderate (33%) to severe (22%). (See Figure 11.2 for severity of impairment for anxiety.) Anxiety disorders are heterogenous, indicating that they comprise a wide range of different disorders. Phobias are the most common anxiety disorder with a prevalence of 10 percent, followed by panic disorder with or without agoraphobia (6%), social anxiety disorder (2.7%), and generalized anxiety disorder (2.2%).[3]

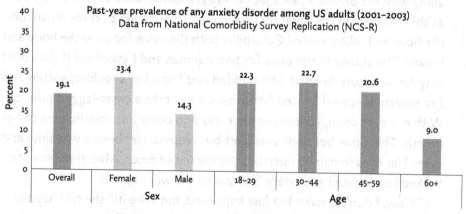

Figure 11.1 Anxiety prevalence among US adults[4]

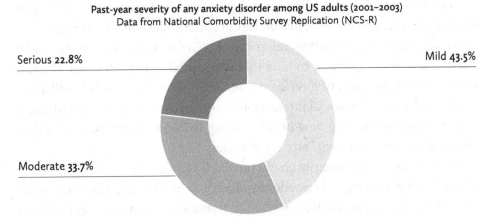

Figure 11.2 Severity of anxiety disorders among US adults[5]

Symptoms of anxiety are a normal reaction to stress and can even be beneficial at times—for example, when we need to respond to something quickly to prevent harm from occurring (slamming on the brakes when a car in front of you stops short unexpectedly). Anxiety disorders, however, differ from normal responses to perceived threats in that they involve excessive fear, worry, or anxiety. Such excessive levels of anxiety can impact daily life in many ways, including high degrees of tension in the body, avoidance behavior (shying away from situations that might trigger symptoms), and panic attacks. Avoidance behavior in particular can lead to problems with job performance, school, and personal relationships.

The experience of anxiety has two main components, the physical (e.g., tension, headaches, shortness of breath) and the emotional (e.g., nervousness, worry, fear, feeling that one is going to die), both of which impact overall cognitive processes, including thinking, decision-making, problem-solving, attention, and new learning.[6] According to the DSM-5, there are six types of anxiety disorders which share two core features: the anxiety is out of proportion to the situation or age-inappropriate, and it hinders the ability to function normally.[7]

Specific phobia is the most common type of anxiety, and it occurs when there is a persistent, excessive fear of a specific object, situation, or activity that causes such distress that sufferers often go to great lengths to avoid the feared stimulus. Such phobias are grouped into major categories such as animal type, natural environment type, situational type, blood-injection-injury type, and "other." The most common type of specific phobia is fear of confined places—including small rooms without windows, elevators, and tunnels—followed by highway driving, water, flying, dogs, animals, insects, thunder, public transportation, injuries involving blood, and dental/medical procedures.[8]

Social anxiety disorder is the second most common type, and as the name suggests, it relates to extreme discomfort in social situations that creates a fear of embarrassment, humiliation, rejection, or being looked down upon in social interactions. It is important to note that with social anxiety disorder, the fear is excessive to the point of interference in daily functioning: people will avoid situations that involve social interactions or only get through them with great anxiety. Fear of meeting new people, eating/drinking in public, and public speaking are common social anxiety disorders.

Panic disorder is primarily characterized by panic attacks, overwhelming physical and psychological episodes in which any or all of the following symptoms occur: heart palpitations, sweating, trembling, chest pain, shortness of breath, dizziness, light-headedness or fainting, fear of choking, tingling or numbness, chills or hot flashes, nausea and gastrointestinal (GI) distress, fear of losing control, and fear of dying. These symptoms can be so severe that sufferers often believe they are having a heart attack or other life-threatening episode and might seek emergency care.

To be diagnosed with a panic disorder, a person must experience a panic attack followed by one month or more of fear that they are going to have more attacks, leading to changes in their behavior (often avoidance of situations) to prevent another attack. Panic attacks can come on unexpectedly or in response to a feared object or situation.

Agoraphobia is next on the list in terms of frequency; it is the fear of being in situations where escape may not be possible, or the fear that having a panic attack might lead to extreme embarrassment. These situations might include being on public transportation, being in enclosed places, being in a crowd, or even simply being outside of one's home.

Generalized anxiety disorder is also common and involves persistent and excessive worry that interferes with normal daily activities. These worries often center around everyday things such as family, health, appointments, or work-related obligations. Such ongoing worry can create both physical and emotional symptoms, including problems with sleep, concentration, and muscle tension.

Finally, there is separation anxiety disorder, which most often develops in childhood and involves excessive fear or anxiety around being separated from loved ones beyond what is age-appropriate, causing problems with daily functioning. A child with separation anxiety may be extremely worried about being parted from the person they love or might even refuse to go out. In some cases, these symptoms can carry through into adulthood.[9]

The causes of anxiety disorder, like depression, are likely due to a combination of genetics, biological and developmental factors, environment, and psychological factors. Anxiety disorders often run in families, suggesting some type of genetic predisposition. Brain imaging and functional studies have shown that neurotransmitters are linked with anxiety, including gamma-aminobutyric acid (GABA), serotonin, and norepinephrine. Environmental impacts, including adverse events in childhood or adulthood, life stressors, and even natural disasters, can also play a role in the development of anxiety disorders.

There is also a learned or behavioral component to anxiety which can get strengthened over time through avoidance behaviors. Researchers first recognized this connection through fear-conditioning experiments on rats and humans by the famous 1920s Russian physiologist Ivan Pavlov and by American psychologist John Watson.[10, 11] There is also a high rate of co-morbidity between depression and anxiety (symptoms of both conditions occur at the same time or sequentially), as more than 50 percent of people with depression also experience some type of anxiety disorder.[12]

TREATMENT FOR ANXIETY

Despite the facts that anxiety is the most prevalent of psychiatric conditions and that it is one of the most responsive to treatment, less than 30 percent of those who suffer from anxiety seek treatment.[13] Treatments for anxiety include psychotherapy with behavioral therapy (used for phobias typically involving exposure to the feared object or situation using guided imagery, progressive desensitization, or flooding), cognitive behavioral therapy to eliminate or reduce automatic anxious thought patterns, talk therapy to explore early developmental and other family dynamics, and medications such as antidepressants, benzodiazepines, and beta blockers. Meta-analysis of different treatments for anxiety shows that the combination of psychotherapy (particularly CBT) and medications yielded a high effect size.[14, 15, 16]

However, side-effects of medications, particularly the traditional anti-anxiety medications (benzodiazepines), can cause potential issues with psychomotor impairment and dependence. In addition, many people are hesitant to seek out mental health support or are limited by the very anxiety that they are struggling with (e.g., agoraphobia/social phobia). As a result, over the last 20 years, there has been an increase in the use of alternative or complementary medicine for treatment of anxiety and other mental health conditions, including relaxation techniques,[17, 18] herbal medicine,[19, 20] yoga,[21] acupuncture,[22] and many others.[23, 24]

RESEARCH ON YOGA FOR ANXIETY

Yoga has been looked at extensively over the past several decades as a possible adjunctive treatment for anxiety. It is a practice that can be done in people's own homes, which makes it much more accessible for people who struggle to leave the house or find that talking to someone about their problems only seems to heighten their anxiety. In addition, because yoga is often practiced at home, it does not require an expensive membership to a studio or gym. A survey in 2012 in the United States indicated that nearly half of US adults who practiced yoga did not actually attend formal classes in a yoga studio or fitness center. Instead, they were practicing at home, either self-led or using online platforms.[25]

There have been several reviews of both the effectiveness and safety of yoga for people with elevated levels of anxiety as well as formal anxiety disorders. These reviews have found that, to date, there is promising but insufficient evidence to support the use of yoga for anxiety. Over the past five years, more randomized control studies have been conducted that have shown that yoga may be beneficial for reducing the intensity of anxiety, as compared to no treatment or other non-medical treatments such as exercise. However, the research is still considered preliminary and further randomized control trials are needed to provide conclusive support for yoga as an effective treatment for anxiety disorders.[26, 27, 28, 29]

Researchers have recently begun to look at specific types of yoga, including different yoga breathing (*pranayama*) practices, and at practice settings, to see if there are additional factors to consider when recommending yoga for anxiety. *Pranayama* has long been considered helpful in treating anxiety. A recent study found that *bhastrika pranayama* (Bellows Breath), which utilizes rapid expirations generated by contraction of the abdominal muscles, significantly reduced anxiety. Furthermore, a functional MRI (fMRI) showed changes in specific areas of the brain following the utilization of this *pranayama* practice. These included areas associated with emotional processing, attention, and awareness, providing key insights into how yoga may be effective in treating anxiety and other mental health conditions.[30] Promising new research also suggests that community yoga, practiced in everyday settings like a gym, can be quite effective in reducing participants' stress and anxiety. Yoga that is inexpensive, easy to access, and with the added benefit of group support can decrease barriers to utilizing yoga on a regular basis for many people.[31]

Researchers have begun to examine the underlying mechanisms of yoga's promising effects on anxiety. They have found that it increases levels of the inhibitory neurotransmitter gamma-aminobutyric acid in the thalamic region of the brain (similar to how anxiety medications target GABA levels and produce an anxiolytic effect).[32, 33] In addition, *pranayama* practices, including coherent breathing, alternate nostril breathing, and *bhastrika* practices, have been shown to shift the sympathetic nervous system activation toward a parasympathetic response via the vagal stimulation that occurs with breath practices.[34, 35, 36]

These findings have been borne out through the use of breath practices and relaxation that have long been a part of various cognitive behavioral treatments for anxiety, particularly panic disorders. Breath work within a yoga practice, especially long slow breathing, helps practitioners to stay calm and focused. *Dirgha* and *ujjayi pranayama* can help individuals stay relaxed within difficult or uncomfortable poses or sensations, essentially keeping the mind focused on the present moment while activating the parasympathetic nervous system. This can produce stress relief even within challenging or uncomfortable sensations.

Through the practice of yoga, individuals can learn how to tolerate stress rather than avoid it—an important skill, given that avoidance often maintains or even strengthens the intensity of an anxiety disorder. Decreasing avoidance to emotional and physical discomfort on the yoga mat could potentially be generalized to day-to-day life experiences and provide individuals with new skills and confidence to manage stressors that would previously have created high levels of anxiety.[37, 38]

Yin yoga can be especially effective in enhancing the parasympathetic nervous system response within gentle and relatively static postures, as well as slowly increasing tolerance for stronger sensations. Several new randomized control trial studies over the past few years have looked at yin yoga specifically as a treatment modality for anxiety.[39, 40] The results are promising, in that they have demonstrated that yin yoga-based interventions can decrease the biomarker plasma adrenomedullin, which is related to an elevated risk for cardiovascular and mental health conditions, including anxiety and other stress-related disorders. Another study suggests that yin yoga coupled with yogic breathing and mindfulness produces greater reductions in anxiety, depression, and sleep as compared to control groups.[41]

In my clinical practice, I have utilized a combination of yin yoga, mindfulness, and psychoeducation to treat many different types of anxiety and have found that this approach can be particularly effective in addressing the physiological arousal that accompanies many anxious conditions, as well as the worrying/rumination that can be so detrimental to people's quality of life. When my clients are anxious, I will often start first with more active practices rather than beginning in a meditation or yin pose. As I described with Cassie, it can be helpful to match a person's current energy level to their yoga practice.

To target anxiety, I will frequently start with some movement and *pranayama* and then move toward a more mindfulness-based practice, integrating yin poses as tolerated. Simple movements might include Breath of Joy, half or full Sun Salutations, or other standing poses such as Dancing Warrior or Horse Stance.

For yin poses, I find that the Kidney/UB series created by Sarah Powers is a very helpful sequence for my clients to practice on a regular basis once they have begun to tolerate longer holding of poses. These poses include forward folds and gentle backbends that are accessible to most individuals, even beginners. Sarah describes how "the Kidney and UB meridian organs' influence on our body-mind is connected with the limbic system housed near the center of the brain." She continues:

> If we also take poses that stimulate the nourishment of the Kidney and UB meridians (that flow through the brain), we accelerate the chemical and attitudinal balance we need. Our practice can be a place where we create positive experiences to store in the limbic system's emotional memory by inviting challenging circumstances (holding a yin pose) while we relax our struggle with whatever emotional difficulty we are facing.[42]

I will often weave in psychoeducation about anxiety, the nervous system, and automatic negative thoughts while clients are holding different shapes to provide an understanding on an intellectual/cognitive level, along with the direct felt experience of the practice using yin inquiry cues about physical sensations in the body.

Anxiety disorders can create a lifelong struggle with uncomfortable physical symptoms including high degrees of tension in the body, excessive worry, and avoidance behavior. Many of my clients have shared how they have spent countless hours in their lives worrying about situations that may not even happen! Yoga has played an increasingly important role in supporting the reduction in anxiety as more and more people seek out alternatives to traditional treatment including anti-anxiety medications. I now regularly rely on teaching a combination of yin yoga, mindfulness techniques, and cognitive behavioral strategies to provide my clients with a toolkit of coping skills to manage their anxiety. I have seen first-hand how these coping skills have transformed their lives by giving them the confidence that they can handle stressful situations by utilizing their own inner wisdom they have discovered through these yoga and meditation practices.

ENDNOTES

1 www.weforum.org/agenda/2019/01/this-is-the-worlds-biggest-mental-health-problem

2 www.nimh.nih.gov/health/statistics/any-anxiety-disorder

3 Shri, R. (2010) 'Anxiety: Causes and management.' *Journal of Behavioral Science, 5,* 1, 100–118. https://s006.tci-thaijo.org/index.php/IJBS/article/view/2205.

4 www.nimh.nih.gov/health/statistics/any-anxiety-disorder

5 www.nimh.nih.gov/health/statistics/any-anxiety-disorder

6 Shri, R. (2010) 'Anxiety: Causes and management.' *Journal of Behavioral Science, 5,* 1, 100–118. https://s006.tci-thaijo.org/index.php/IJBS/article/view/2205.

7 American Psychiatric Association (2013) *Diagnostic and Statistical Manual of Mental Disorders* (5th ed.) (DSM-5). Arlington, VA: APA.

8 https://www.psychiatry.org/patients-families/anxiety-disorders/what-are-anxiety-disorders

9 American Psychiatric Association (2013) *Diagnostic and Statistical Manual of Mental Disorders* (5th ed.) (DSM-5). Arlington, VA: APA.

10 Garakani, A., Mathew, S.J., and Charney, D.S. (2006) 'Neurobiology of anxiety disorders and implications for treatment.' *Mount Sinai Journal of Medicine, 73,* 7, 941–949.

11 Bandelow, B., Michaelis, S., and Wedekind, D. (2017) 'Treatment of anxiety disorders.' *Dialogues in Clinical Neuroscience, 19,* 2, 93–107.

12 Mineka, S., Watson, D., and Clark, L.A. (1998) 'Comorbidity of anxiety and unipolar mood disorders.' *Annual Review of Psychology, 49,* 1, 377–412.

13 Shri, R. (2010) 'Anxiety: Causes and management.' *Journal of Behavioral Science, 5,* 1, 100–118. https://s006.tci-thaijo.org/index.php/IJBS/article/view/2205.

14 Shri, R. (2010) 'Anxiety: Causes and management.' *Journal of Behavioral Science, 5,* 1, 100–118. https://s006.tci-thaijo.org/index.php/IJBS/article/view/2205.

15 Garakani, A., Mathew, S.J., and Charney, D.S. (2006) 'Neurobiology of anxiety disorders and implications for treatment.' *Mount Sinai Journal of Medicine, 73,* 7, 941–949.

16 Bandelow, B., Michaelis, S., and Wedekind, D. (2017) 'Treatment of anxiety disorders.' *Dialogues in Clinical Neuroscience, 19,* 2, 93–107.

17 Kessler, R.C., Soukup, J., Davis, R.B., *et al.* (2001) 'The use of complementary and alternative therapies to treat anxiety and depression in the United States.' *American Journal of Psychiatry, 158,* 2, 289–294.

18 Shri, R. (2010) 'Anxiety: Causes and management.' *Journal of Behavioral Science, 5,* 1, 100–118. https://s006.tci-thaijo.org/index.php/IJBS/article/view/2205.

19 Kessler, R.C., Soukup, J., Davis, R.B., *et al.* (2001) 'The use of complementary and alternative therapies to treat anxiety and depression in the United States.' *American Journal of Psychiatry, 158,* 2, 289–294.

20 Shri, R. (2010) 'Anxiety: Causes and management.' *Journal of Behavioral Science, 5,* 1, 100–118. https://s006.tci-thaijo.org/index.php/IJBS/article/view/2205.

21 NIH (2009) 'Complementary, Alternative, or Integrative Health: What's In a Name?' National Center for Complementary and Alternative Medicine, National Institutes of Health. https://www.nccih.nih.gov/health/complementary-alternative-or-integrative-health-whats-in-a-name.

22 Cauffield, J.S. (2000) 'The psychosocial aspects of complementary and alternative medicine.' *Pharmacotherapy, 20,* 11, 1289–1294.

23 Cauffield, J.S. (2000) 'The psychosocial aspects of complementary and alternative medicine.' *Pharmacotherapy, 20,* 11, 1289–1294.

24 NIH (2009) 'Complementary, Alternative, or Integrative Health: What's In a Name?' National Center for Complementary and Alternative Medicine, National Institutes of Health. https://www.nccih.nih.gov/health/complementary-alternative-or-integrative-health-whats-in-a-name.

25 Cramer, H., Ward, L., Steel, A., Lauche, R., Dobos, G., and Zhang, Y. (2016) 'Prevalence, patterns, and predictors of yoga use: Results of a US nationally representative survey.' *American Journal of Preventative Medicine, 50*, 2, 230–235.

26 Cramer, H., Lauche, R., Anheyer, D., *et al.* (2018) 'Yoga for anxiety: A systematic review and meta-analysis of randomized controlled trials.' *Depression and Anxiety, 35*, 9, 830–843.

27 Kirkwood, G., Rampes, H., Tuffrey, V., Richardson, J., and Pilkington, K. (2005) 'Yoga for anxiety: A systematic review of the research evidence.' *British Journal of Sports Medicine, 39*, 12, 884–891.

28 Hofmann, S.G., Andreoli, G., Carpenter, J.K., and Curtiss, J. (2016) 'Effect of hatha yoga on anxiety: A meta-analysis.' *Journal of Evidence-Based Medicine.* doi: 10.1111/jebm.12204.

29 Novaes, M., Palhano-Fontes, F., Onias, H., *et al.* (2020) 'Effects of yoga respiratory practice (Bhastrika pranayama) on anxiety, affect, and brain functional connectivity and activity: A randomized controlled trial.' *Frontiers in Psychiatry, 11*, article 467.

30 Novaes, M., Palhano-Fontes, F., Onias, H., *et al.* (2020) 'Effects of yoga respiratory practice (Bhastrika pranayama) on anxiety, affect, and brain functional connectivity and activity: A randomized controlled trial.' *Frontiers in Psychiatry, 11*, article 467.

31 Maddux, R., Daukantaite, D., and Tellhed, U. (2018) 'The effects of yoga on stress and psychological health among employees: An 8- and 16-week intervention study.' *Anxiety, Stress, & Coping 31*, 2, 121–134.

32 Streeter, C.C., Jensen, J.E., Perlmutter, R.M., *et al.* (2007) 'Yoga asana sessions increase brain GABA levels: A pilot study.' *Journal of Alternative and Complementary Medicine, 13*, 4, 419–426.

33 Streeter, C.C., Whitfield, T.H., Owen, L., *et al.* (2010) 'Effects of yoga versus walking on mood, anxiety, and brain GABA levels: A randomized controlled MRS study.' *Journal of Alternative and Complementary Medicine, 16*, 11, 1145–1152.

34 Novaes, M., Palhano-Fontes, F., Onias, H., *et al.* (2020) 'Effects of yoga respiratory practice (Bhastrika pranayama) on anxiety, affect, and brain functional connectivity and activity: A randomized controlled trial.' *Frontiers in Psychiatry, 11*, article 467.

35 Streeter, C.C., Whitfield, T.H., Owen, L., *et al.* (2010) 'Effects of yoga versus walking on mood, anxiety, and brain GABA levels: A randomized controlled MRS study.' *Journal of Alternative and Complementary Medicine, 16*, 11, 1145–1152.

36 Brown, R.P., and Gerbarg, P.L. (2005) 'Sudarshan Kriya Yogic breathing in the treatment of stress, anxiety, and depression: Part I—Neurophysiological model.' *Journal of Alternative and Complementary Medicine, 11*, 4, 711–717.

37 Maddux, R., Daukantaite, D., and Tellhed, U. (2018) 'The effects of yoga on stress and psychological health among employees: An 8- and 16-week intervention study.' *Anxiety, Stress, & Coping 31*, 2, 121–134.

38 Schmidt, N.B., Woolaway-Bickel, K., Trakowski, J., *et al.* (2000) 'Dismantling cognitive-behavioral treatment for panic disorder: Questioning the utility of breathing retraining.' *Journal of Consulting and Clinical Psychology, 68, 3*, 417–424.

39 Daukantaite, D., Tellhed, U., Maddoux, R., Svensson, T., and Melander, O. (2018) 'Five-week yin yoga-based interventions decreased plasma adrenomedullin and increased psychological health in stressed adults: A randomized controlled trial.' *PLoS One, 13*, 7.

40 Tellhed, U., Daukantaite, D., Maddux, R., Svensson, T., and Melander, O. (2019) 'Yogic breathing and mindfulness as stress coping mediate positive health outcomes of yoga.' *Mindfulness, 10*, 2703–2715.

41 Tellhed, U., Daukantaite, D., Maddux, R., Svensson, T., and Melander, O. (2019) 'Yogic breathing and mindfulness as stress coping mediate positive health outcomes of yoga.' *Mindfulness, 10*, 2703–2715.

42 Powers, S. (2008) *Insight Yoga.* Boulder, CO: Shambhala Publications, p.35.

Chapter 12

YIN YOGA FOR PTSD AND COMPLEX TRAUMA

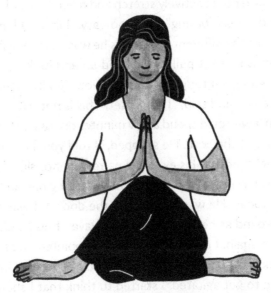

Shoelace provides a safe container to explore hip, back, and abdominal stimulation

My client, Jack, was a friendly, gregarious, and handsome 60-year-old man. He owned his own company and a large home in the suburbs that he shared with his wife and two dogs. Jack came to me because he had started taking yoga classes at the local gym and found that it was helpful for managing what he called "stress." He thought that having some individual sessions might help him to get "better" at yoga.

During our first yoga therapy session, Jack seemed upbeat and eager to practice. Since he had some experience with yoga, I suggested we start with a grounding meditation followed by three-part breath (*dirgha pranayama*). We sat together and he seemed quite comfortable with these two initial practices.

I had him move into warm-ups and then flowed through Sun Salutations. He was strong and athletic and quickly found a fast-paced rhythm to do his Sun Salutations. I asked him if he could slow down, and he easily held poses for up to ten breaths without breaking a sweat. I asked him if he had ever done any yin poses before. He shook his head and said that he was eager to try something new. I had him take Butterfly—my usual "test" to see if a client has any challenges with longer holdings and how they might encounter this type of quieter experience.

Jack seemed a bit restless at first as he took the shape. I asked him if he needed any props to support him or provide him with more ease. He shook his head but seemed irritated. "This is easy," he said, and then pulled himself forward, reaching for his feet. I asked him if he could try to soften and round his shoulders rather than actively stretch and reach forward. He sighed loudly and said that this was "boring" and "too easy." I invited him to focus on his breath and notice the different sensations he was experiencing. He was clearly tuning me out as he kept pulling his head up and looking toward the door, looking at his watch, and adjusting his position. Finally, after about four minutes, he popped up and said, "I am all set. This is not what I am looking for."

I asked him if we could spend a few minutes discussing how he was feeling and the purpose of the pose. He snapped, "I told you, I am all set." Jack's face had turned bright red and his eyes had narrowed into slits. I saw that he was getting increasingly upset. I apologized for upsetting him and thanked him for his hard work today. He was heading for the door as I was speaking, and he did not turn around as he gave me a small wave of his hand. Well, I thought, I won't see him again. I immediately felt disappointed and like I had failed in some way. Jack was enjoying the practice and as soon as I introduced him to yin, he seemed to get agitated. I started to think that I should have just had him stick with more active poses, but then I realized that I would not have seen some potential triggers that might be a key to helping him manage his stress.

Unexpectedly, Jack called and left me a long message at 5 a.m. on my voice mail. He explained that he was very sorry for getting so upset and that he liked the yoga very much. He went on to say that he has a bad temper and he does not know what gets him so upset, but this has been a chronic issue. He listed several areas of his life in which he was struggling with his anger, including his marriage, his work, and estrangement from his son. He asked to come back and have another session.

We met the following week and I decided to review some ideas for practice with Jack before we started an actual sequence. I asked him questions about what he liked and what was challenging about our class last week. He stated that "I feel strong when I do Sun Salutations. I love the feeling of moving and breathing. But that Butterfly pose, you kept me there forever. I hated it. I felt trapped. Stuck. Like there was nowhere to go. I just felt this overwhelming urge to get up and leave."

I asked Jack if he had ever felt that way before. He nodded. Then he shared that he had had a single mother who was verbally, emotionally, and physically abusive toward him and his younger brother throughout their childhood. He suffered many beatings until he was about 12 years old. He had grown taller that year and he told his mother that if she put her hands on him one more time, he would hit her back. The beatings stopped, but she continued to call him "stupid," "a loser," "a joke of a son."

Jack left home at age 16 and never returned. He entered the army at age 18, went on to college, and continued on to earn his MBA. However, he frequently had nightmares about his childhood, waking up thinking that his mom was chasing him with a belt or throwing things at him. He became extremely defensive and angry if he perceived that other people were criticizing him. His first marriage ended in divorce after only one year due to his temper. He did not have much contact with his young son because "I did not know how to be a father."

Jack began to cry as he shared how much he regretted that he could not control his anger and how he has pushed people away. He shared that he had had suicidal thoughts in the past, especially after he had had an anger episode. I asked Jack if he ever talked to a therapist. He reported that he had seen a psychiatrist at the Veterans Affairs (VA) hospital and was admitted on one occasion to the inpatient ward after "losing it" in the emergency room when he was not able to get treatment right away for acute GI distress. He did not want to take medications because "I don't like the side-effects," he said, and that he largely managed day to day through intense exercise and working 12-hour days and avoiding being around people. I asked Jack what he was treated for, and he said that they told him that he had post-traumatic stress disorder (PTSD) from his childhood. He said that he hated that this made him feel weak and like a loser (mirroring what his mother said to him many years ago).

We began our second session together by doing coherent breathing for two minutes together. My goal was to help him develop a more balanced and regulated nervous system. He followed along and kept his eyes open and seemed to tolerate the slower breath. Since he really enjoyed the flow practice last week, I invited him to select a series of warm-ups that felt best in his body. He quietly moved through a sequence of Cat/Cow and Extended Table, and moved into Sun Salutations and Warriors. He was breathing heavily now and sweat began pouring off him. I asked him to see how it would feel to gently slow down and stay in a pose for 10 to 20 breaths. I reminded him that he could come out of the pose at any time and take another shape or just relax. I gave him a few options—Butterfly, Caterpillar, Sphinx, or Seal pose—showing him each one. He selected Seal pose, enjoying the intensity of the backbend and the effort and engagement of his upper body as he stayed in the pose.

After about two minutes, he eased his way down into Sphinx pose on his own. His breath slowed down, and his eyes remained open, but softer, for the next few minutes. I stayed quiet and had him just breathe and notice any sensations. I invited him to try Frog next with the option to go into Wide-Knee Child. He chose again to take a more gentle pose after two minutes in the more intense Frog, easing into Wide-Knee Child, looking more relaxed. We continued to do this yang/yin experiment by first doing a more intense yang pose followed by a softer yin variation with Sleeping Swan (upright/yang), followed by Sleeping Swan (reclining/yin), Shoulder Stand (yang), followed by Supported Bridge (yin), and then a brief constructive rest at the end. I remained largely quiet, providing only posture cues and a few gentle reminders to notice his sensations along with complete permission to choose to move at any time.

After the formal session, we spent a few minutes debriefing. Jack told me that he felt something release in him during the yin poses, but he needed to feel the muscular engagement and strong sensations first "so I could tolerate the softer ones." When I asked him what he meant by softer ones, his eyes filled with tears and he said, "You know, like grief, sadness, stuff I have pushed away for so long." We worked on some distress tolerance skills that he could utilize during practice and off the mat as well, including radical acceptance for his experience, self-compassion for his distress, and grounding using the senses if he is getting very dysregulated.

Jack reliably came to our yoga therapy sessions for the next several years! He ended up becoming a yoga teacher himself and even teaching yin yoga to veterans at the VA hospital. He said that the biggest takeaways for him during his early yin yoga experiences was how hard it was to stop moving and just feel his emotions and physical sensations, but that once he was able to break through and meet his pain, something shifted and allowed him to begin to process the full range of his feelings. He still isolates from others when he is distressed to avoid even the potential for having an anger outburst as he is terrified of lashing out and hurting others as he did in the past. However, he goes to his yoga mat often and uses a combination of Vinyasa and flow followed by a steady dose of yin and finds this to be a reset if he is struggling emotionally.

Post-traumatic stress disorder is a serious psychological condition that often develops after exposure to a traumatic event or multiple events. It is most common among combat veterans, survivors of wars and natural disasters, and victims of violence. While going through trauma is relatively common (between about 50 and 60 percent of adults have experienced at least one significant trauma in their lives), the actual number of people who develop PTSD is much smaller by comparison (between 7–8% of adults).

Women have a higher rate than men, nearly double (10% of women develop PTSD sometime in their lives compared to about 4% of men). (See Figure 12.1 for prevalence breakdown by gender and age.) Women are more likely to experience sexual assault and child sexual abuse, while men are more likely to experience accidents, physical assaults, combat, or disaster, or witness a death or serious injury. (See Table 12.1 for prevalence of PTSD by type of traumatic event.) Severity of impairment indicates how challenging this condition is, with over two-thirds of those diagnosed with PTSD suffering from moderate to serious impairment (33% moderate; 36% serious), and another one-third with mild impairment. [1, 2] (See Figure 12.1 for severity of impairment for PTSD.)

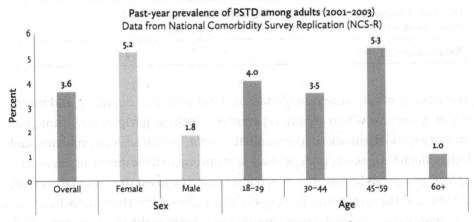

Figure 12.1 Prevalence of PTSD among adults[3]

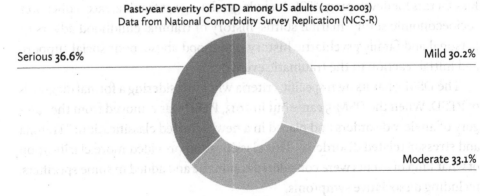

Figure 12.2 Severity of impairment among US adults[4]

Table 12.1 PTSD statistics by trauma[5]

Traumatic event	Examples of trauma	Percentage of people who will develop PTSD
Sexual relationship violence	Rape, childhood, sexual abuse, intimate partner violence	33%
Interpersonal-network traumatic experience	Unexpected death of loved one; life-threatening illness of a child	30%
Interpersonal violence	Childhood physical abuse or witnessing interpersonal violence, physical assault, being threatened by violence	12%
Exposure to organized violence	Refugee, kidnapped, civilian in war zone	3%
Participation in organized violence	Combat exposure, witnessing death/ serious injury or discovered dead bodies, accidently or purposely caused death or serious injury	11%
Other life-threatening traumatic events	Life-threatening motor vehicle collision, toxic chemical exposure	12%
Natural disaster victims		3.8%

The severity of impairment depends on the chronicity, frequency, and intensity of symptoms which are often persistent, including frightening thoughts, memories, and flashbacks of the traumatic event, as well as sleep problems, and feeling detached, numb, or depressed. It is normal to have upsetting memories or feeling anxious and overwhelmed after being exposed to a traumatic event. However, if the symptoms develop early (usually within three months of the traumatic event), or persist over time (at least one month), they are more likely to develop into PTSD. However, sometimes the symptoms only start years later. Risk factors for developing PTSD include gender, age at trauma, race, education, socioeconomic status, marital status, history of trauma, childhood adversity, personal and family psychiatric history, childhood abuse, poor social support, and initial reaction to the traumatic event.[6]

The DSM-5 has its own specific criteria when considering a formal diagnosis of PTSD. When the DSM-5 came out in 2013, PTSD was removed from the category of anxiety disorders and placed in a newly created classification: "Trauma and stressor-related disorders." This classification provided more clarification of what kind of events were considered traumatic and added in some specifiers, including dissociative symptoms.

While the recognition of PTSD as being part of a separate classification was widely valued with this new addition, several pioneers in the field of trauma, including Bessel van der Kolk, were unhappy that developmental trauma disorder was not considered a "formal diagnosis" in this iteration of the DSM-5. "Developmental trauma disorder" refers to alterations in affect, behavioral regulation, interpersonal problems, dissociative symptoms, and somatization that occur in children and adolescents who have been subjected to complex trauma.[7] A new task force created as the DSM-5 was being developed in the early 2000s (led by van der Kolk) conducted research with traumatized children and found that while only about 25 percent of children who were exposed to multiple or prolonged trauma met the criteria for PTSD, they still had significant problems regulating emotions, including poor impulse control, aggression, dissociation, and poor self-esteem. Their main argument for including developmental trauma in the next iteration of the DSM was that understanding the etiology of trauma, especially early repeated childhood trauma, can help clinicians better understand the number of psychosocial risk factors that may develop especially when the formal PTSD diagnosis is *not* met.

The creators (many of whom were based in academic rather than clinical settings) of the DSM-5 ultimately did not allow this new diagnosis because they felt that the range of symptoms proposed was too broad and would supersede many other diagnoses. However, many clinicians who work with this population insist that this expanded definition of trauma is critical to understanding the impact of childhood trauma such as emotional and physical abuse, neglect, and maltreatment.[8, 9, 10] Further, the data support a high psychiatric co-morbidity in clients with PTSD (an estimated 88% of people with PTSD had at least one co-occurring diagnosis). About half of all of those diagnosed with PTSD have three or more conditions, including depression, anxiety, and substance abuse.[11]

In my own clinical work, I have found that utilizing the framework provided by the developmental trauma classification is extremely important in understanding the complex emotional, interpersonal, and behavioral presentations of my clients. Many of my clients have come to me with diagnoses of PTSD, borderline personality disorder, bipolar disorder, and major depression. While they may have met the criteria for these conditions, treating just the symptoms of one or more of these complex issues without examining and beginning to unpack childhood developmental trauma had often created a cycle of failed treatment with repeated hospitalizations, multiple medications, and inability to move forward with age-appropriate developmental milestones (finding satisfaction in jobs, relationships, and self).

Because only their classic PTSD symptoms like flashbacks or avoidance behaviors had been addressed, many of my clients continued to suffer from the abuse of their past in terms of their ability to regulate emotions, maintain solid relationships, and have adequate self-esteem. The practices I suggest throughout this chapter are designed for people who have been diagnosed with PTSD as well as those who have experienced significant developmental trauma.

TREATMENT FOR PTSD

According to the American Psychological Association (APA), there are two main types of treatment for PTSD: psychotherapy and pharmacotherapy.[12] Based on the research, there are four types of psychotherapy (all of which are forms of cognitive behavioral therapy) that are strongly recommended:

- Cognitive behavioral therapy (CBT): Focus is on the relationship between thoughts, feelings, and behaviors. Method involves changing patterns of behaviors, thoughts, and feelings that lead to problematic functioning.
- Cognitive processing therapy (CPT): Focus is on modifying and changing unhelpful beliefs specifically related to the trauma. Method involves helping to create a new understanding of the traumatic event to reduce negative impact on current life.
- Cognitive therapy (CT): Focus is on modifying the pessimistic evaluations and actual memories of the trauma. Method involves interrupting the distressing behavioral and thinking patterns associated with the trauma that have been interfering with daily life.
- Prolonged exposure therapy (PE): Focus is on approaching trauma-related memories, feelings, and experiences. Method involves facing memories that have previously been avoided and learning that these memories are not dangerous once they are processed.[13]

In addition to those described above, the US Department of Veteran Affairs recommends eye movement desensitization and reprocessing (EMDR) therapy as highly effective. EMDR involves bilateral stimulation (focusing on a bilateral back-and-forth movement such as fingers, sound, or light touch) while at the same time calling the trauma to mind, which supports the processing of the trauma to reduce its negative impact on the person.

Medications have received only conditional recommendation by the APA and VA for treatment of PTSD, all in the antidepressant category, including sertraline, paroxetine (these two are the only ones recommended by the FDA, along with fluoxetine and venlafaxine).[14, 15] Recent studies have suggested that most medications for PTSD have only shown a small benefit as compared to placebo.[16, 17] As a result, psychotherapy is generally considered to be the "gold standard" for treatment of PTSD. Efficacy of psychotherapy has shown more promise in different meta-analyses, especially some of the specific trauma-focused interventions described above.[18, 19]

However, many people cannot tolerate the intensity of some of these trauma-focused treatments, which can cause them to prematurely terminate treatment before the benefits have fully been experienced, or can even increase emotional distress. Dropout rates and non-responsiveness to treatment are also often quite high for other trauma therapies, especially among those individuals suffering from complex trauma (30 to 60%).[20, 21, 22, 23]

As a result of the challenges with traditional treatments for PTSD, many people are interested in the use of complementary and alternative treatments, including yoga and other mind-body approaches.[24, 25, 26] Bessel van der Kolk and colleagues have postulated that traditional PTSD treatments have such a high rate of incomplete responding because other important domains are not included, such as emotional dysregulation, spirituality, and negative beliefs about meaning and purpose in life.[27, 28] Researchers and yoga practitioners have been investigating how yoga might be effective in the treatment of PTSD and other traumas, particularly in terms of emotion regulation. There has been ample research over the past three decades supporting the use of yoga and meditation to calm the mind and body and increase life satisfaction.[29, 30, 31, 32]

RESEARCH ON YOGA FOR PTSD

Yoga is now utilized with growing frequency to treat PTSD and trauma survivors in a variety of settings, including VA clinics and hospitals, trauma treatment centers, and outpatient sites across the world. David Emerson, one of the pioneers in leading yoga for trauma survivors, created trauma-sensitive yoga (TSY) as part of a best-practice approach to teaching yoga for PTSD. Through his clinic at the Trauma Center Yoga Program at the Justice Resource Institute, Emerson and colleagues developed yoga-teaching principles and practices to create a safe and healing environment for trauma survivors. These principles include creating a space that makes participants feel safe and comfortable (avoiding triggers like exposed windows, loud noises, etc.), using trauma-sensitive yoga poses appropriate for the diverse population of trauma survivors (e.g., military veterans vs. adult survivors of sexual trauma), providing options for all postures, teaching cues with awareness of a warm and nonjudgmental attitude, pace, avoiding physical assists, and the use of invitatory language rather than commands.[33]

Research on the efficacy of this TSY approach has shown that this form of yoga is effective with women with trauma, particularly those that have suffered interpersonal trauma/violence, and may reduce depression and anxiety that is co-occurring along with PTSD. The studies have also shown increased participant satisfaction and increased likelihood to continue a yoga practice in contrast to some of the traditional psychological treatments, where retention is often quite poor.[34] In terms of other dimensions of healing from trauma, researchers have investigated TSY in terms of personal growth and perceived changes in symptoms following a course of treatment. Themes that were found in participants' responses after completing a ten-week TSY program included gratitude, compassion, relatedness, acceptance, centeredness, and empowerment.[35] Other populations using TSY, including women veterans who experienced military sexual trauma, have also been shown to have a positive impact, including quicker symptom improvement and retention than alterative trauma-focused psychotherapy.[36]

The underlying mechanisms of yoga have been examined in terms of how yoga postures and meditation might reduce some of the key psychoneuroimmunology of PTSD, including autonomic dysregulation, activation of the hypothalamic-pituitary-adrenal (HPA) axis, and inflammatory activation response. Researchers have postulated that yoga can reduce cortisol levels, influence several different neurotransmitters, and increase neurotrophic factors that can reduce overall inflammation. These changes can effectively counteract or reduce the impact of stress, anxiety, and negative mood.[37, 38]

While these studies have shown promise in terms of symptom improvement and longer commitment to treatment, there are very few actual randomized control studies and the sample sizes of many studies are quite limited. A recent meta-analysis showed that there is only "low quality evidence that yoga interventions could be an effective, acceptable and safe intervention for PTSD."[39] Therefore, there is a strong need for ongoing research and high-quality studies to confirm some of the promising effects that many of these smaller studies have shown and to support the underlying mechanisms proposed by researchers to explain how yoga can effectively reduce PTSD symptoms.

YIN YOGA FOR PTSD

Yin yoga may be a particularly effective form of yoga to reduce the impact of some symptoms that are unique to PTSD and the long-lasting effects of traumatic stress on the body. van der Kolk states that most effective treatments for PTSD include practices that increase tolerance to physical sensations in the body, reduce or regulate physiological arousal in the body, and involve learning how to create effective actions in the body to counteract the physical helplessness that often occurs in PTSD.[40]

In my experience, yin yoga can be one of the first therapeutic types of body-based practices wherein participants with trauma can regulate how much sensation they are experiencing, and incrementally increase tolerance to physical sensations in a gradual manner so as not to overwhelm the nervous system and to create a sense of self-efficacy and control over one's own body.

I like to introduce yin yoga poses in a careful and thoughtful way when working with someone who reports having a history of trauma or a PTSD diagnosis. Initially, I find shapes that are accessible, easily modifiable, and do not place clients in a vulnerable position (e.g., Butterfly or other poses that might feel exposing) so that they can begin to work in the three qualities that van der Kolk suggested: increase tolerance, regulate arousal, and create effective action. I will often shorten the duration of the pose to 60–90 seconds or have the participant decide when they want to come out of the pose to increase their sense of control over their own body. I like to do the poses together with my client at the same time so that they don't feel like I am staring at them or creating an expectation of performance. I like to speak aloud for each of the steps coming in and out of a pose and add in brief explanations so that there is a sense of understanding and reassurance about the purpose and method of what we are doing.

The use of *pranayama* has been very helpful for my clients while exploring different yin poses. It creates an anchor for their minds to focus on and can reduce overall arousal. We will start with simple mindfulness of breathing using the visualization of a *cellular breath* to help to stay present and grounded. I ask my clients to imagine that the whole body is actually breathing as every cell receives oxygen from the breath. I will then introduce *dirgha pranayama* (3-part breath) with the *ujjayi* sound which can be very grounding and stabilizing.

Another element of practice that I will frequently include is a yoga *nidra* meditation at the end or beginning of the practice with descriptive instructions in the beginning and ample modifications offered (eyes open, sitting up, shortened practice). I also often select poses from both the Kidney/UB sequence and the Liver/Gallbladder sequence to address nervous system regulation.

Sarah Powers says, "When we have a liver chi imbalance, we have a propensity for uneven, irregular emotions; chronic anger; explosive impulsivity; a defense of personal boundaries; and awkward social behavior."[41] Enabling clients to experience waves of emotions, even anger, within the safety of a yin pose can help provide a sense of hope that these feelings will not last forever and provide them with the confidence that they can handle their own reactions.

I find that one of the keys to working with clients with trauma both as a yoga therapist and a clinician is to consciously tune in to my own internal responses to ensure I am creating a sense of grounding and stability in my guidance. By tuning in to the interoceptive cues in my body, including physical sensations, feelings, and emotions, I am able to attend mindfully to potential triggers for the client and adjust my guidance accordingly. For example, when I start to notice sympathetic nervous system arousal occurring in my own body by observing my breath shorten, my heart rate quicken, and my chest tighten, I might recognize that I am teaching too quickly or creating a pressured environment for the client. To adjust, I will slow down my teaching, take a mindful pause, and check in with the client to see how they are feeling. By keeping my attention tuned in to my own experience while at the same time monitoring the client, I can likely avoid triggering the client or creating an extremely unpleasant situation that might cause harm. If my client does get dysregulated, I provide options for grounding through the use of the senses, coherent breathing, or simply taking a mindful pause and encouraging the use of journaling, walking, or other soothing options preferred by the client. Overall, I have found that while there can be moments of dysregulation like what occurred with Jack, I have also seen so many clients with PTSD and complex trauma discovering more peace and joy in their lives through the healing power of yoga and mindfulness.

ENDNOTES

1   www.nimh.nih.gov/health/statistics/post-traumatic-stress-disorder-ptsd.shtml
2   www.ptsd.va.gov/understand/common/common_adults.asp
3   www.nimh.nih.gov/health/statistics/post-traumatic-stress-disorder-ptsd.shtml
4   www.nimh.nih.gov/health/statistics/post-traumatic-stress-disorder-ptsd.shtml
5   Kessler, R.C., Rose, S., Koenen, K.C., et al. (2014) 'How well can post-traumatic stress disorder be predicted from pre-trauma risk factors? An exploratory study in the WHO World Mental Health Surveys.' World Psychiatry: Official Journal of the World Psychiatric Association (WPA), 13, 3, 265–274.
6   Sareen, J., Erickson, J., Medved, M.I., et al. (2013) 'Risk factors for post-injury mental health problems.' Depression and Anxiety, 30, 4, 321–327.
7   Sareen, J., Erickson, J., Medved, M.I., et al. (2013) 'Risk factors for post-injury mental health problems.' Depression and Anxiety, 30, 4, 321–327.

8   Schmid, M., Petermann, F., and Fegert, J.D. (2013) 'Developmental trauma disorder: Pros and cons of including formal criteria in psychiatric diagnostic systems.' *BMC Psychiatry, 13*, 3, 1471–244X.

9   Farina, B., and Liotti, G. (2013) 'Does a dissociative psychopathological dimension exist? A review on dissociative processes and symptoms in developmental trauma spectrum disorders.' *Clinical Neuropsychiatry, 10*, 11–18.

10 Farina, B., Liotti, M., and Imperatori, C. (2019) 'The role of attachment trauma and disintegrative pathogenic process in the traumatic-dissociative dimension.' *Frontiers in Psychology, 10*, 933.

11 Kessler, R.C., Sonnega, A., Bromet, E., Hughes, M., and Nelson, C.B. (1995) 'Posttraumatic stress disorder in the National Comorbidity Survey.' *Archives of General Psychiatry, 52*, 12, 1048–1060.

12 American Psychological Association (2021) 'PTSD treatments.' www.apa.org/ptsd-guideline/treatments.

13 American Psychological Association (2021) 'PTSD treatments.' www.apa.org/ptsd-guideline/treatments.

14 American Psychological Association (2021) 'PTSD treatments.' www.apa.org/ptsd-guideline/treatments.

15 US Department of Veterans Affairs (2020) 'PTSD: National Center for PTSD.' www.ptsd.va.gov/understand_tx/tx_basics.asp.

16 Hoskins, M., Pearce, J., Bethell, A., *et al.* (2015) 'Pharmacotherapy for post-traumatic stress disorder: Systematic review and meta-analysis.' *British Journal of Psychiatry, 206*, 2, 93–100.

17 Cipriani, A., Williams, T., Nikolakopoulou, A., *et al.* (2017) 'Comparative efficacy and acceptability of pharmacological treatments for post-traumatic stress disorder in adults: A network meta-analysis.' *Psychological Medicine 2017*, 1–10.

18 Lee, D.J., Schnitzlein, C.W., Wolf, J.P., Vythilingam, M., Rasmusson, A.M., and Hoge, C.W. (2016) 'Psychotherapy versus pharmacotherapy for posttraumatic stress disorder: Systematic review and meta-analysis to determine first-line treatment.' *Depression and Anxiety, 33*, 9, 792–806.

19 Bisson, J.I., Roberts, N.P., Andrew, M., Cooper, R., and Lewis, C. (2013) 'Psychological therapies for chronic post-traumatic stress disorder (PTSD) in adults.' *Cochrane Database of Systematic Reviews, 12*, CD003388.

20 Kline, A.C., Cooper, A.A., Rytwinksi, N.K., and Feeny, N.C. (2018) 'Long-term efficacy of psychotherapy for posttraumatic stress disorder: A meta-analysis of randomized controlled trials.' *Clinical Psychology Review, 59*, 30–40.

21 Kessler, R.C., Sonnega, A., Bromet, E., Hughes, M., and Nelson, C.B. (1995) 'Posttraumatic stress disorder in the National Comorbidity Survey.' *Archives of General Psychiatry, 52*, 1048–1060.

22 D'Andrea, W., and Pole, N. (2012) 'A naturalistic study of the relation of psychotherapy process to changes in symptoms, information processing, and physiological activity in complex trauma.' *Psychological Trauma: Theory, Research, Practice, and Policy, 4*, 4, 438–446.

23 Bradley, R., Greene, J., Russ, E., *et al.* (2005) 'A multidimensional meta-analysis of psychotherapy for PTSD.' *American Journal of Psychiatry, 162*, 214–227.

24 Wynn, G.H. (2015) 'Complementary and alternative medicine approaches in the treatment of PTSD.' *Current Psychiatry Reports, 17*, 8, 600.

25 Kim, S.H., Schneider, S.M., Kravitz, L., Mermier, C., and Burge, M.R. (2013) 'Mind-body practices for posttraumatic stress disorder.' *Journal of Investigative Medicine, 61*, 5, 827–834.

26 Cramer, H., Anheyer, D., Saha, F., and Dobos, G. (2018) 'Yoga for posttraumatic stress disorder: A systematic review and meta-analysis.' *MBC Psychiatry, 18*, 72, 1–9.

27 van der Kolk, B.A., Stone, L., West, J., *et al.* (2014) 'Yoga as an adjunctive treatment for posttraumatic stress disorder: A randomized controlled trial.' *Journal of Clinical Psychiatry, 75*, 6, e559–e565.

28 Jindani, F., and Fatha Singh Khalsa, G. (2015) 'A journey to embodied healing: Yoga as a treatment for post-traumatic stress disorder.' *Journal of Religion & Spirituality in Social Work: Social Thought, 34,* 394–413.

29 Sarang, P., and Telles, S. (2006) 'Effects of two yoga-based relaxation techniques on heart rate variability (HRV).' *International Journal of Stress Management, 13,* 4, 460–475.

30 Benson, H., Alexander, S., and Feldman, C.L. (1975) 'Decreased premature ventricular contractions through use of the relaxation response in clients with stable ischemic heart-disease.' *Lancet, 2,* 380–382.

31 Miller, J.J., Fletcher, K., and Kabat-Zinn, J. (1995) 'Three-year follow-up and clinical implications of a mindfulness meditation-based stress reduction intervention in the treatment of anxiety disorders.' *General Hospital Psychiatry, 17,* 3, 192–200.

32 Reibel, D.K., Greeson, J.M., Brainard, G.C., and Rosenzweig, S. (2001) 'Mindfulness-based stress reduction and health-related quality of life in a heterogeneous client population.' *General Hospital Psychiatry, 23,* 4, 183–192.

33 Emerson, D., Sharma, R., Chaudhry, S., and Turner, J. (2009) 'Trauma-sensitive yoga: Principles, practice, and research.' *International Journal of Yoga Therapy, 19,* 123–128.

34 Nolan, C. (2016) 'Bending without breaking: A narrative review of trauma-sensitive yoga for women with PTSD.' *Complementary Therapies in Clinical Practice, 24,* 32–40.

35 West, J., Liang, B., and Spinazzola, J. (2017) 'Trauma sensitive yoga as a complementary treatment for posttraumatic stress disorder: A qualitative descriptive analysis.' *International Journal of Stress Management, 24,* 2, 173–195.

36 Kelly, U., Haywood, T., Segell, E., and Higgins, M. (2021) 'Trauma-sensitive yoga for post-traumatic stress disorder in women veterans who experienced military sexual trauma: Interim results from a randomized controlled trial.' *Journal of Alternative and Complementary Medicine, 27,* 1, S45–S59.

37 Balasubramaniam, M., Telles, S., and Doraiswamy, P.M. (2012) 'Yoga on our minds: A systematic review of yoga for neuropsychiatric disorders.' *Frontiers in Psychiatry, 3,* 117.

38 Kelly, U., Evans, D.D., Baker, H., and Noggle Taylor, J. (2018) 'Determining psycho-neuroimmunologic markers of yoga as an intervention for people diagnosed with PTSD: A systematic review.' *Biological Research for Nursing, 20,* 3, 343–351.

39 Cramer, H., Anheyer, D., Saha, F., and Dobos, G. (2018) 'Yoga for posttraumatic stress disorder: A systematic review and meta-analysis.' *MBC Psychiatry, 18,* 72, 1–9.

40 van der Kolk, B.A. (2006) 'Clinical implications of neuroscience research in PTSD.' *Annals of the New York Academy of Sciences, 1071,* 277–293.

41 Powers, S. (2008) *Insight Yoga.* Boulder, CO: Shambhala Publications, p.58.

Chapter 13

YIN YOGA FOR TRAUMATIC BRAIN INJURY

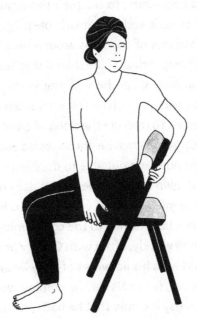

Seated Twist provides an accessible, gentle, and refreshing movement for the spine

When I first met Todd, he was in a wheelchair at a rehabilitation hospital following a traumatic brain injury that had occurred six months earlier as a result of a motorcycle accident. He was accompanied by his young wife Christy, who was clearly caring and invested in her husband's care. Todd was 24 years old, tall, thin, and very intelligent. He was just starting to walk again with the use of a walker, with significant left-sided weakness due to the location of his brain injury which impacted his right hemisphere primarily. His speech was a bit slowed but was clear and articulate. He was funny, insightful, and motivated to keep improving.

Todd was interviewing me to see if he wanted me to become part of his team as he transitioned back into the community to live with his wife. He asked me about my perspective on brain injury recovery and the types of cognitive services I could provide for him. I shared with him that I believe that every brain injury survivor is unique, bringing their own personal strengths and weaknesses, and I don't use one specific modality, but instead utilize different approaches to help.

I asked him if he was interested in any mind-body approaches and his warm brown eyes lit up. He had first begun meditating in college; he also loved being out in nature and engaging in vigorous physical exercise, including running and mountain climbing. Christy became tearful as she described her husband's life before the accident. I could see how much she loved her husband and how much grieving she had been doing to see their promising life together so dramatically altered. Christy reviewed the remarkable progress he had made since his accident, but she had lots of concerns around his physical, cognitive, and emotional functioning going forward. She shared that Todd often got "flooded" by his emotions, particularly when he was angry—he would have bouts of yelling, swearing, and crying. He often felt embarrassed after one of these episodes but felt powerless to manage the flood of emotions. Todd interjected that it had been so frustrating when he encountered something that he could easily do in the past and now was not able to do, even the simplest things like using a bathroom on his own or remembering his daily routine.

Todd decided to hire me, and I was very happy to be part of his ongoing rehabilitation team. Once he returned to the community to live with Christy, I started meeting with him weekly, often with Christy present, or with the caregiver who helped Todd with his activities of daily living, to review the highs and lows of the past week, set goals for the coming week, and troubleshoot challenges in his day-to-day life now that he had returned to the community.

During those early sessions, Todd was very cheerful, making jokes and telling stories about his life prior to his accident. It was hard to get him to talk much about his struggles in the present moment and he would frequently resort to showing me things on his phone like pictures, scores on brain games, or reminiscing about his college days.

After a few months, I began to gently challenge Todd to share more about his feelings. This quickly created an intense reaction in him. He started yelling and swearing, saying, "I want my life back. I hate my brain injury." Christy rushed into the room, saying, "Calm down, Todd," which only seemed to enrage Todd more. He began throwing things and yelling. I asked Christy to leave the room and began to breathe slowly and rhythmically in a quiet, but audible way. After about one minute, Todd quieted. He took my nonverbal cues and began to breathe with me. We sat that way for about ten minutes just breathing, and I watched his face relax and his body ease. Afterward, he shared that when he got flooded, it was as if there were two Todds—one on each shoulder. One was the old Todd who was active, athletic, and had his whole life ahead of him. The other Todd was brain-injured, living at home with his parents, and felt hopeless. When he got flooded, it felt like a war between the two Todds.

Week after week, I worked with Todd on different mindfulness techniques to address this flooding. We utilized the STOP sign (stop, take a breath, observe, and proceed), DBT skills like DEAR MAN and radical acceptance, and compassion practices. Todd was able to use these techniques when he was relaxed, even recalling the acronyms and what they stood for. However, when he was flooded he struggled to remember any techniques.

Meanwhile, I had become involved in a program called LoveYourBrain (LYB) Yoga,[1] which offered community-based yoga classes for traumatic brain injury survivors. Using a structured six-week format, the curriculum centered on adaptive practices, including meditation, asana, and pranayama, along with group support through different topic discussions each week. The adaptations included providing slow, simple, and repeating directions, creating a safe place, monitoring the position of the body, especially head and neck, demonstrating the poses, utilizing props, and ensuring the yoga space was adequate.[2]

I became a certified LYB instructor and had a six-week series in my local yoga studio. Initially, I did not think that Todd was up to the yoga practice, particularly because he still had some difficulty with walking independently (he was now using a cane to ambulate) and I thought it might be hard for him to get up and down off the floor. I met with Todd and Christy, and we reviewed the website and the yoga practices that were available online.

Todd was excited right away by the idea of the LoveYourBrain yoga class. He had not done any physical activity aside from physical therapy and the pool, and he loved the idea of doing more practices in the body that would "help me push myself." Christy was concerned about whether some of the poses would be frustrating for Todd but agreed he could participate provided she could accompany him.

Todd came to the initial session and interacted well with the other brain injury survivors. I watched him as he smiled, greeting his peers with a warm hello, and introduced himself. He was poised and had great energy. How-ever, things abruptly shifted for Todd as we began the yoga practice. Almost immediately, I heard Todd complaining to Christy that he could not see me and did not know what I was saying. He moved to a closer spot, but he was becoming agitated.

I led the class through some gentle warm-ups, and I saw Todd stop midway through the first set and shake his head. He was trying to remain quiet, but his voice began to amplify. "I can't do this. I hate my body. This was a mistake." The group continued the practice but shared supportive encouragement for Todd. This only seemed to make things worse. He began to cry—the first time I had seen him in tears after nearly a year of therapy. Christy and I surrounded him, and I placed a bolster under his knees and blanket under his head and encouraged him to breathe just like we had been practicing. He started to settle and his breathing quieted. I asked him to just remain in this relaxed position as the class went on. He could practice meditation or tune out, whatever would be most helpful.

Todd stayed in this position for about ten minutes. Then, out of the corner of my eye, I saw him begin to stretch and move his body gently from side to side, coming into a Reclining Twist. Christy placed a bolster under his knees, and he stayed on each side for a minute or two. I went over and quietly asked him if he might want to try a Supported Bridge using his bolster. He agreed and while the rest of the class was starting to transition to standing, Todd took a Supported Bridge and continued to focus on his breath.

I continued to teach the class, and every few minutes I would check to see if Todd wanted to stay in his pose or take another shape. He agreed to try a reclining Butterfly for his final pose, with two blocks underneath each knee and a bolster supporting his back. His eyes were closed, and his breath was steady. The rest of the class eventually joined Todd in *Savasana*.

At the end of the class, we formed a circle to explore how the practice was and discuss whether there were any silver linings to having a brain injury. Todd raised his hand and spoke first. He said, "I was so active before my TBI, I could climb mountains, run for hours, play soccer. Since my TBI, I have been at war with my body. It does not move the way I want it to. Today, I hated this practice. I hated Tracey for suggesting it. I was ready to give up. Then, I saw you guys and how you kept going. That helped me not totally lose it. Tell you the truth, I kind of liked it at the end, especially the twist. My back feels really good."

The group applauded warmly, and the rest of the participants shared their experiences. At the end of the class, I walked over to Todd and Christy.

> They looked hopeful, the way they had when I first met them both in the rehabilitation hospital. Christy said, "I am so proud of Todd. He was able to calm down and actually experience frustration and success." I patted Todd on the shoulder and said, "You are now a yogi," and put my hands up to my heart in prayer position and bowed. "*Namaste.*"
>
> His eyes danced and his smile was bright. "*Namaste.*"

A traumatic brain injury (TBI) is caused by a sudden external insult to the head (a blow, jolt, bump, gunshot wound, or fall) that disrupts the normal functioning of the brain. This is considered a primary brain injury, in that the injury is completed at the time of the impact. In contrast, a secondary brain injury refers to one that evolves over a period of time, sometimes hours to even days after a primary brain injury. It can include chemical, tissue, and blood vessel changes that can lead to further damage; it can be very serious, potentially even leading to death.

Closed brain injuries are the most common type of traumatic brain injury, occurring when there is a rapid forward-and-backward, shaking movement of the brain causing bruising, tearing, and shearing of brain tissue and blood vessels (referred to as a coup-countercoup injury, as the damage occurs directly to the site of the impact and then as the brain jolts backwards, it can hit the skull on the opposite or "countercoup" side). Closed brain injuries are most commonly caused by motor vehicle accidents and falls. Penetrating brain injuries are open head injuries that occur when there is a break in the skull, such a bullet piercing the brain.[3]

Not all head injuries are "brain injuries." Many of us have fallen off a bike and hit our heads or, as toddlers, hit our heads on a table and did not sustain any brain damage at all. The severity of a TBI can range from mild to severe, with the majority being mild (these are referred to as concussions). The four main measures of severity used to classify a TBI include the duration of loss of consciousness; post-traumatic amnesia (PTA); which refers to the period of memory loss following an injury until the person can continuously recall information again; brain imaging (CT scan or MRI); and a test called the Glasgow Coma Scale (GCS), which is a measure of a person's level of consciousness and neurological functioning post brain injury using a scale of 1–15.

Different classification schemas for TBIs have been utilized without any universally recognized system. The American Congress of Rehabilitative Medicine's definition of mild traumatic brain injury and the Mayo classification system for traumatic brain injury severity were developed to more reliably categorize TBI severity.

The Mayo system has been shown to have a stronger accuracy than other systems. It has three main classifications, including Moderate to Severe TBI (definite), Mild TBI (probable), and Symptomatic TBI (possible). Classification systems such as the Mayo system can be a helpful starting point for clinicians to predict recovery and rehabilitation outcomes, and to provide important information to the brain injury survivor and family members in terms of potential supports needed in the short term and the long term. (See Table 13.1 for the Mayo classification system of TBI severity.) Misclassification can occur especially with some of the more subjective or difficult-to-determine indicators such as PTA, which can be inaccurate especially if a client was heavily medicated at the time of injury.[4, 5, 6]

In addition, there has been significant controversy around mild TBI (MTBI) because sometimes individuals who sustain even very mild traumatic brain injuries have ongoing symptoms that can be quite impactful in terms of day-to-day functioning. As a result, it is important to recognize that the term *mild TBI* is in fact only referring to the initial severity of the brain injury, not to the prognosis or long-term impact of the injury.

Table 13.1 Mayo classification system of TBI severity[7]

Classification	Loss of consciousness	Post-traumatic amnesia	Glasgow Coma Scale	Imaging
Possible TBI based on one or more of the following symptoms: blurred vision, confusion, dizziness, headache, nausea	Possible	Possible	N/A	N/A
Mild TBI	Less than 30 minutes	Less than 24 hours	N/A	Indicating depressed, basilar, or linear skull fracture (dura intact)
Moderate to severe TBI	30 minutes or more	24 hours or greater	Worst GCS full score in first 24 hours is less than 13	Hematoma, contusion, hemorrhage

TBI STATISTICS

TBI is a major public health problem in the United States and across the world. According to the Centers for Disease Control and Prevention (CDC), the most recent statistics published (in 2019) indicated that about 2.87 million TBI-related emergency visits, hospitalizations, and deaths occurred in the United States in one year alone (2014). Further, the number of these emergency visits have increased significantly, by approximately 53 percent, between 2006 and 2014. The leading cause of TBI (and likely contributing to the increasing numbers of TBI over the last decade) are falls among the elderly, at 52 percent. The second leading cause is motor vehicle accidents at 20 percent.

TBI is a major cause of death and disability in the United States. The CDC reports that an average of 155 people in the United States die each day from injuries that include a TBI (that's 56,800 people, including 2529 children). When people survive following a TBI, they may have deficits that persist for days, weeks, or years, potentially causing lifelong disabilities. Studies indicate that approximately 5.3 million people in the United States (2% of the population) are suffering from long-term disabilities as a result of TBI, with direct and indirect annual costs of more than 56 billion dollars.[8, 9, 10]

TBI is known as the "silent epidemic" because while some symptoms appear right away (e.g., nausea or vomiting), many problems are not immediately apparent and may not be obvious until the person attempts to return to everyday life. TBI symptoms usually fall into three main categories: physical, cognitive, and emotional/behavioral. Physical complaints include headache, fatigue, insomnia, dizziness, tinnitus, light and sound sensitivity, and more severe deficits that may occur in moderate to severe TBIs, including paralysis or hemiparalysis, oral-motor problems (difficulty with speech/swallowing), incontinence, and muscle tone problems. Cognitive complaints include memory problems—especially short-term—and difficulties with attention and/or concentration, higher-level reasoning, and problem-solving/executive functioning. Emotional/behavioral issues often involve depression, anxiety, irritability, mood swings, and anger/rage. Even relatively mild brain injuries can cause "post-concussive symptoms" that can last three to six months and sometimes longer.[11]

Many individuals with traumatic brain injuries have some type of ongoing physical, cognitive, and/or psychological impairment even when they have had a good recovery from their initial injury. There is strong preliminary evidence suggesting that TBI may increase the likelihood of developing a psychiatric disorder, particularly depression and anxiety.[12] There are many factors that play a role in developing psychiatric disorders following TBI, including the location of the injury, injury severity, premorbid psychiatric symptoms (history of mental health problems in the past or relevant family history), pre-injury substance use, and individual psychosocial factors.[13]

As a result, there has been considerable research over the past several years around the co-morbidity between TBI and psychiatric disorders. The rates of psychiatric disorders after TBI vary depending on several factors, including the severity and location of the brain injury, pre-existing conditions, and overlap with other medical conditions that can produce similar symptoms (insomnia, fatigue, lack of interest). Other factors, including mental fatigue and chronic pain, which can impact individuals with traumatic brain injury, can cause irritability, sensitivity to stress, concentration difficulties, and emotional instability. Depression is the most common psychiatric condition among patients with TBI, with a prevalence ranging from 18 to 60 percent depending on the study, followed by anxiety, with a prevalence of 10 to 30 percent. Patients with TBI are also at increased risk for bipolar disorder, obsessive-compulsive disorder, PTSD, schizophrenia/psychotic disorders, and personality disorders.[14, 15, 16, 17]

TBI REHABILITATION

The development of psychological impairment is one of the best predictors of overall post-injury adjustment, even ten years post-TBI.[18] I discovered this early on in my career, when I began working with brain injury survivors during my internship at the Miami VA hospital. Many of the clients that were referred to me had a significant brain injury but were being referred to the psychology clinic because they were experiencing emotional or behavioral issues even years after their initial injury.

The veterans would report high levels of depression, frustration, anger management issues, and PTSD long after they had sustained a brain injury. They would be confused about why they did not feel like themselves even though they could walk, talk, and "seemed normal." Many had tried traditional treatments, including medications and psychotherapy, but this often made their condition worse, not better. Their frustration and hopelessness increased my commitment to discovering new and innovative ways of working with TBI survivors.

Over the last 20 years, I have continued to work with different brain-injury populations, including acute inpatient brain injury rehabilitation, day treatment, and individual outpatient assessment and treatment of traumatic brain injury survivors. In each of these settings, I have been struck by the significant treatment barriers for TBI survivors, especially those experiencing psychiatric conditions impacting emotion regulation and behavioral control.

In early phases of rehabilitation (within days to weeks of the brain injury), individuals with moderate to severe brain injuries often have significant behavioral problems (e.g., agitation, impulsivity, mood lability), causing problems in settings where the primary emphasis is on physical rehabilitation, not emotional/ psychiatric treatment. This could lead to brain injury clients being inappropriately placed in other settings, like nursing homes or psychiatric units, or simply being discharged to home too early because they are a management problem. If they are sent to mental health treaters or psychiatry units, brain injury clients are often unable to participate fully in traditional psychotherapy treatments due to cognitive deficits. Further, psychiatric medication may exacerbate aspects of the brain injury and cause increasing problems with emotional regulation. As was the case for many of the veterans I treated in my early career, receiving care in inappropriate settings and taking psychiatric medications without ongoing careful monitoring can create a cycle of failed treatments or interrupt true healing and recovery.

In later stages of rehabilitation (after the first one to three months following an injury), returning to the community or attempting to resume life as it was before the injury can further exacerbate psychological distress. The outside environment, including responsibilities with family, finances, and daily life, can quickly become overwhelming, especially when an individual is still struggling with physical, cognitive, and emotional symptoms. As a result, psychiatric problems can intensify several months or even years after the initial injury.

In addition, personality changes that often go undetected early in the rehabilitation process become more pronounced as individuals return to their communities and families. Typical personality changes occur in the following domains: reduced social perceptiveness, reduced control/self-regulation, problems with initiation and planning, emotional changes (apathy, jocularity, mood swings), difficulty learning from experience, disinhibition, self-focused, poor insight, and child-like or dependent personality traits.[19, 20] Many of these changes, along with problems with attention and concentration, are associated with frontal lobe injuries. It is not uncommon for depression to increase rather than decrease over time, depending on psychosocial factors and environment; some studies report the prevalence of increased depression to be as high as 60 percent at the seven-year mark as compared to 20–30 percent during the first year.[21]

Treatment strategies for traumatic brain injury and psychiatric disorders usually center around medications and traditional cognitive behavioral therapy. The management of psychiatric disorders most often starts with managing agitation and/or aggression, which can lead to violence or self-harm if not treated. However, medications used to treat aggression are often sedating and can increase confusion and agitation, leading to a paradoxical effect for patients.

For this reason, non-pharmacological treatments are often preferred when possible, to avoid the cycle of failed treatments that some of my veterans reported. Typically, behavioral and cognitive behavioral treatments are considered to be the first choice for many clients with challenging behaviors, as they are widely known to be helpful for depression and anxiety.[22] However, in my experience, clients with brain injuries often have difficulty participating in these therapies, which require significant attention/concentration or memory and the ability to utilize acquired skills in daily life. There have been very few randomized control studies to establish any particular type of therapy or medication as the treatment of choice. As a result, in treating TBI patients who suffer from psychiatric disorders a comprehensive approach must be considered, including a combination of medication, psychotherapy, and skill building.

My early training in rehabilitation included inpatient TBI programs with many professionals working in multidisciplinary teams, usually led by a physician (physiatrist, internist, or psychiatrist), with physical therapists, occupational therapists, speech and language pathologists, recreational therapists, and social workers (in addition to neuropsychologists like me). We would meet weekly or sometimes even daily to review patients' goals, progress, and discharge planning. Hearing from each professional, I would learn something new about the patients' capacities or the challenges they were experiencing which would inform the work I was doing as a neuropsychologist.

Sometimes we would work together in a session—we called it "tag-teaming"—when we thought the client would benefit from the intersection of our services. For example, one of my clients would get very tearful and cry during her physical therapy sessions, so I came to a session and worked with her on distress tolerance and positive self-talk while she was doing her walking and strengthening exercises. Then we would take a break and have a conversation about movies, handsome actors, and her hopes and dreams for the future. By the end of the session, she was able to push through more challenging exercises and felt a sense of accomplishment.

My role as a neuropsychologist changed significantly when I moved to outpatient rehabilitation. In this setting, I was sometimes the only person working with the client if they were coming in for therapy or neuropsychological assessment. I often had only limited medical history about the person's TBI and other issues. They would sometimes come with a family member which would be helpful, but sometimes they would come alone or with an aide from a nursing home who did not have any specific history to provide. These clients needed many services but were often unsure of how to get them. Sometimes, their TBI was many years ago and they were only there because one of their doctors thought it would be helpful for them to have an evaluation.

Right at the time that I started doing outpatient TBI services, the state of

Connecticut started a program using a federal Medicaid community-based model called the "Acquired Brain Injury (ABI) waiver." The waiver referred to the ability to "waive" some of the typical Medicaid requirements to allow more individuals to live in the community and receive services in their homes, to "relearn, improve or retain the skills needed to live successfully in the community."[23] The program was self-directed in that the participant is the employer who manages the direction of their program, including hiring, firing, and establishing the roles and duties of their support staff. Each program included a neuropsychologist who would support the participant and lead the team to ensure services were being appropriately provided, goals were effective, and the client's needs were being met.

My first client on this program, Beth, had been living in a congregate living space for over a decade, and this would be the first time she would be living on her own in the community. I was working at an outpatient clinic and was charged with setting up a "program" for her in the community, so she could live safely and maximize her independence. I was excited about this new program and thrilled to be working on creating a better quality of life for TBI clients. I went to see her new living space, a lovely, accessible first-floor apartment. Beth was sitting in the kitchen in a power wheelchair when I arrived. She was nonverbal due to her TBI and used a small computer to spell out her thoughts and pressed a button to share out loud what she had transcribed. She had an aide with her who sat quietly in the other room, looking through a magazine.

As soon as I introduced myself, Beth pressed "play" and a message began in a computerized mechanical voice. "I have been institutionalized for many years. I want to be more independent. I want to have meaning and purpose in my life." She nodded and smiled as I reassured her that we would be working together to help her make these goals come to fruition.

Inwardly, I felt a deep fear come over me. I had no idea where to begin. What supports would she need to reach these goals? I looked through a short discharge summary from her congregate living setting, and saw that she needed assistance in all her activities of daily living (ADLs), including bathing, dressing, transfers, and toileting, and some supports in her higher-level independent activities of daily living (IADLs) in terms of budgeting, money management, shopping, and cooking. In addition, she had a history of major depression with suicidal ideation. The fear deepened in my stomach. This was going to be much harder than I imagined.

I quickly recognized that although I was supposed to be a team leader,

Beth was actually the one who needed to drive the plan. Her hopes, dreams, and goals needed to be front and center to make this program work the way it was designed. Beth's motivation and her team's understanding of her goals and needs would be the key to whether this program would succeed.

Based on the work of Edward Deci and Richard Ryan, human motivation can be understood by the self-determination theory (SDT), which examines the needs of a person through the lens of *competency, autonomy,* and *relatedness.* If these core needs are met, natural growth and intrinsically motivated behavior will ensue. Intrinsic motivation is more sustainable than extrinsically based rewards that can fade in their potency over time.[24] I recognized this early on in my work with brain injury clients when we utilized extrinsic rewards like food/coffee/trips to try to motivate them to do their rehabilitation exercises. At first, they would work hard to earn the reinforcer, but over time it became harder and harder to find reinforcers that could sustain the effort required to complete sometimes painful routines.

In Daniel Pink's book *Drive,* he describes three keys to intrinsic motivation: *autonomy, mastery,* and *purpose.*[25] In thinking about Beth, I recognized how important it was going to be to help her find intrinsic motivation through finding a sense of autonomy and mastery, even though she needed assistance in some of the most basic self-care tasks and for her to seek out a community where she could feel part of something larger that held meaning and purpose for her. To begin this program would require a team approach, including the right professionals across different disciplines, to move from a rehabilitation approach, which is often time-limited and missing key life-enhancing qualities, to a *habilitation* approach which emphasizes living life with what you have and maximizing purpose and meaning. These habilitation team members might include not only the typical ones found in most hospitals and clinics (physical therapist, occupational therapist, speech and language pathologist, and neuropsychologist and traditional medical providers such as a physiatrist and behavioral neurologist), but also mental health providers such as a marriage and family therapist, a psychiatrist, and a substance abuse counselor, and finally, holistic practitioners such as a yoga therapist, mindfulness teacher, and life coach.

I was fortunate that Beth was open to exploring new and innovative ideas for her new life in her own apartment. Over the 20 years that I have been working with Beth, she has participated in advocacy groups for people with disabilities, submitted testimony to the state legislature on funding and health care, mastered new speech and communication devices so that she can converse more quickly in "real time" with others, and flown on a plane by herself to Florida to visit her family.

Beth has ups and downs with her mood and has required antidepressant medications along with ongoing supportive therapy since her program began. She struggles with hiring and firing of her staff and gets frustrated quickly when she perceives that her staff are not meeting her needs. In my weekly work with her, she has continued to work on emotion regulation and impulsivity. Over the past few years, Beth has even started to do some chair yoga with me. These holistic practices, meditation and now yoga, have been helpful with increasing Beth's sense of competency and her social connections. For many TBI survivors, comprehensive treatment using both traditional and alternative approaches may be an important part of a paradigm change from short-term rehabilitation to long-term habilitation.

YOGA AND TBI REHABILITATION

Research around integrative treatments for TBI such as mindfulness has grown over the past two decades.[26, 27, 28] Most of these studies have focused on the milder spectrum of TBIs and there has been less research with mixed or more severe TBI populations which may be due to the difficulty in implementing these approaches with those that are more cognitively challenged and may have difficulty practicing mindfulness. Modifications such as shortening the duration of meditation, using simpler language, having visual aids, and more repetition of topics may support a wider group of TBI survivors.[29]

More recently, yoga for different TBI populations, including both military and non-military, has been explored, with an emphasis on adaptation of physical movements along with cultivation of acceptance and mindful awareness. Benefits were found in several areas, including mental fatigue, improved respiratory functioning, balance, endurance, sleep quality, mental health, physical health, and quality of life.[30, 31, 32, 33] Two recent meta-analyses showed quite promising results in utilizing yoga for TBI populations, with the data supporting robust improvements in fatigue and depression along with psychological and physical adjustment and overall quality of life. Like the research on mindfulness, the yoga studies were conducted with mild TBI populations, which might limit generalizability across the full range of traumatic brain injury.[34, 35] But overall, the latest research on TBI and yoga suggests that yoga brings additional benefits to mindfulness-based interventions alone in the areas of fatigue, respiratory functioning, sleep quality, balance, and quality of life.

In my personal experience working with a full range of TBI survivors with mild to severe injuries, yoga can play an important role in an overall habilitation program, particularly when integrating yin yoga poses into the practices. Yin yoga is accessible to many TBI survivors because the poses can be modified, props can be utilized, and shapes can be done bilaterally or unilaterally depending on range of motion. In addition, the directions are simple and straightforward with ample opportunity to repeat as needed during each pose. There are no complex sets of movements linked together as in traditional Vinyasa or Hatha yoga practices, making it much less complicated to direct. Finally, yin poses can be done without having to transition from floor to standing or standing to floor. Instead, they can be done in one area, floor-based if possible, or even in a wheelchair or a bed.

This last piece is important for clients like Todd, who was able to do many of the floor-based poses but had great difficulty going from floor to standing. By staying on the floor, he was able to complete practices with full independence rather than needing one or even two people to help him transition from floor to standing, which was both disruptive and distressing to him when he participated in my class.

In the habilitative approach, exploring themes during the poses—including resilience, meaning, competence, relatedness, agency, self-compassion, and community—can be particularly supportive to TBI clients. Each theme can serve as an individual inquiry in each pose, or they can be explored as a group of habilitative themes to create a sense of ongoing capacity growing from class to class over time. Since TBI survivors often struggle with impulsivity, attention/concentration, and frustration tolerance—which are part of executive functioning from a cognitive perspective— my TBI clients often report that staying focused for a period of time in a pose and building on it slowly also increases their capacity to focus on tasks in other areas of life.

If a client is particularly restless, sometimes I will start with as little as 30 to 60 seconds in a pose. I will utilize simple counting of the breath out loud and provide support and encouragement, to allow them to sense the desire to move or talk and try to delay it by a few breaths.

The first few times I led yin poses to a class of TBI survivors, I found that there was a lot of conversation! Many of them were comfortable with me and were used to saying out loud any thoughts that came to them in the moment. Some laughed, told jokes, or complained about discomfort. Instead of saying, "Shhh...you are not supposed to talk in a yoga class," I would gently acknowledge their statements, thank them for sharing their experiences, and then invite the class to settle back into the breath. I wanted to create a sense of belonging rather than shaming, correcting, or ignoring. Over time, I would encourage them to stay silent for longer periods if they could, or to raise their hand if they wanted me to come over to assist them. Group programs such as LYB yoga and individual yoga therapy sessions for TBI survivors have continued to expand in popularity because they fit so beautifully within a habilitative approach. Through yoga, I have been able to witness my clients grow and expand their physical and emotional capacity to live their lives to the fullest.

ENDNOTES

1   www.loveyourbrain.com/yoga

2   Chauhan, N., Zeller, C., and Donnelly, K. (2020) 'Best practices for adapting and delivering community-based yoga for people with traumatic brain injury in the United States and Canada.' *International Journal of Yoga Therapy, 30,* 1, 89–101.

3   Brain Injury Association of America (2016) *The Essential Brain Injury Guide* (5th ed.). Fairfax, VA: Brain Injury Association of America.

4   Malec, J.F., Brown, A.W., Leibson, C.L., *et al.* (2007) 'The Mayo classification system for traumatic brain injury severity.' *Journal of Neurotrauma, 24,* 9, 1417–1424.

5   Friedland, D., and Hutchinson, P. (2013) 'Classification of traumatic brain injury.' *Advances in Clinical Neuroscience and Rehabilitation.* https://acnr.co.uk/2013/07/classification-of-traumatic-brain-injury.

6   McAllister, T., and Arciniegas, D. (2002) 'Evaluation and treatment of postconcussive symptoms.' *NeuroRehabilitation, 17,* 265–283.

7   Malec, J.F., Brown, A.W., Leibson, C.L., *et al.* (2007) 'The Mayo classification system for traumatic brain injury severity.' *Journal of Neurotrauma, 24,* 9, 1417–1424.

8   World Health Organization (1992) *International Statistical Classification of Diseases and Related Health Problems* (10th ed.). Geneva, Switzerland: World Health Organization.

9   Centers for Disease Control and Prevention (2019) *Surveillance Report of Traumatic Brain Injury-Related Emergency Department Visits, Hospitalizations, and Deaths—United States, 2014.* Centers for Disease Control and Prevention, US Department of Health and Human Services.

10 Van Reekum, R., Cohen, T., and Wong, J. (2000) 'Can traumatic brain injury cause psychiatric disorders?' *Journal of Neuropsychiatry and Clinical Neurosciences, 12,* 316–327.

11 McAllister, T., and Arciniegas, D. (2002) 'Evaluation and treatment of postconcussive symptoms.' *NeuroRehabilitation, 17,* 265–283.

12 Van Reekum, R., Cohen, T., and Wong, J. (2000) 'Can traumatic brain injury cause psychiatric disorders?' *Journal of Neuropsychiatry and Clinical Neurosciences, 12,* 316–327.

13 Silver, J., Kramer, R., Greenwald, S., and Weismann, M. (2001) 'The association between head injuries and psychiatric disorders: Findings from the New Haven NIMH Epidemiologic Catchment Area Study.' *Brain Injury, 15,* 11, 935–945.

14 Silver, J., Kramer, R., Greenwald, S., and Weismann, M. (2001) 'The association between head injuries and psychiatric disorders: Findings from the New Haven NIMH Epidemiologic Catchment Area Study.' *Brain Injury, 15,* 11, 935–945.

15 Schwarzbold, M., Diaz, A., Martins, E.T., *et al.* (2008) 'Psychiatric disorders and traumatic brain injury.' *Neuropsychiatric Disease Treatment, 4,* 4, 797–816.

16 Osborn, A.J., Mathias, A.K., and Fairweather-Schmidt, K. (2014) 'Depression following adult, non-penetrating traumatic brain injury: A meta-analysis examining methodological variables and sample characteristics.' *Neuroscience and Biobehavioral Reviews, 47,* 1–15.

17 Soo, C., and Tate, R. (2007) 'Psychological treatment for anxiety in people with traumatic brain injury.' *Cochrane Database of Systematic Reviews, 3,* 1–24.

18 Johansson, B., Bjuhr, H., and Rönnbäck, L. (2012) 'Mindfulness-based stress reduction (MBSR) improves long-term mental fatigue after stroke or traumatic brain injury.' *Brain Injury, 26,* 13–14, 1621–1628.

19 Fleminger, S. (2008) 'Long-term psychiatric disorders after traumatic brain injury.' *European Journal of Anaesthesiology, 25* (Suppl 42), 123–130.

20 Hibbard, M.R., Uysal, S., Kepler, K., Bogdany, J., and Silver, J. (1998) 'Axis I psychopathology in individuals with traumatic brain injury.' *Journal of Head Trauma Rehabilitation, 13,* 24–39.

21 Hibbard, M.R., Uysal, S., Kepler, K., Bogdany, J., and Silver, J. (1998) 'Axis I psychopathology in individuals with traumatic brain injury.' *Journal of Head Trauma Rehabilitation, 13,* 24–39.

22 Fleminger, S. (2008) 'Long-term psychiatric disorders after traumatic brain injury.' *European Journal of Anaesthesiology, 25* (Suppl 42), 123–130.

23 https://portal.ct.gov/-/media/Departments-and-Agencies/DSS/Health-and-Home-Care/Community-Options/Acquired-Brain-Injury-Program.pdf

24 Deci, E.L., and Ryan, R.M. (2000) 'The "what" and "why" of goal pursuits: Human needs and the self-determination of behavior.' *Psychological Inquiry, 11,* 227–268.

25 Pink, D. (2009) *Drive.* New York: Riverhead Books.

26 Johansson, B., Bjuhr, H., and Rönnbäck, L. (2012) 'Mindfulness-based stress reduction (MBSR) improves long-term mental fatigue after stroke or traumatic brain injury.' *Brain Injury, 26,* 13–14, 1621–1628.

27 Bédard, M., Felteau, M., Marshall, S., Cullen, N., *et al.* (2014) 'Mindfulness-based cognitive therapy reduces symptoms of depression in people with a traumatic brain injury: Results from a randomized controlled trial.' *Journal of Head Trauma Rehabilitation, 29,* E13–E22.

28 Bédard, M., Felteau, M., Mazmanian, D., Fedyk, K., *et al.* (2003) 'Pilot evaluation of a mindfulness-based intervention to improve quality of life among individuals who sustained traumatic brain injuries.' *Disability and Rehabilitation: An International, Multidisciplinary Journal, 25,* 722–731.

29 Bédard, M., Felteau, M., Marshall, S., Cullen, N., *et al.* (2014) 'Mindfulness-based cognitive therapy reduces symptoms of depression in people with a traumatic brain injury: Results from a randomized controlled trial.' *Journal of Head Trauma Rehabilitation, 29,* E13–E22.

30 Johansson, B., Bjuhr, H., and Rönnbäck, L. (2012) 'Mindfulness-based stress reduction (MBSR) improves long-term mental fatigue after stroke or traumatic brain injury.' *Brain Injury, 26,* 13–14, 1621–1628.

31 Schmid, A.A., Miller, K.K., Van Puymbroeck, M., and Schalk, N. (2016) 'Feasibility and results of a case study of yoga to improve physical functioning in people with chronic traumatic brain injury.' *Disability and Rehabilitation: An International Multidisciplinary Journal, 38,* 914–920.

32 Silverthorne, C., Khalsa, S.B., Gueth, R., DeAvilla, N., and Pansini, J. (2012) 'Respiratory, physical, and psychological benefits of breath focused yoga for adults with severe traumatic brain injury (TBI): A brief pilot study report.' *International Journal of Yoga Therapy, 22,* 47–51.

33 Combs, M.A., Critchfield, E.A., and Soble, J.R. (2018) 'Relax while you rehabilitate: A pilot study integrating a novel, yoga-based mindfulness group intervention into residential brain injury rehabilitation program.' *Rehabilitation Psychology, 63,* 2, 182–193.

34 Silveira, K., and Smart, C.M. (2020) 'Cognitive, physical, and psychological benefits of yoga for acquired brain injuries: A systematic review of recent findings.' *Neuropsychological Rehabilitation, 30,* 7, 1388–1407.

35 Acabchuk, R.L., Brisson, J.M., Park, C.L., Babbott-Bryan, N., Parmelee, O.A., and Johnson, B.T. (2020) 'Therapeutic effects of meditation, yoga, and mindfulness-based interventions for chronic symptoms of mild traumatic brain injury: A systematic review and meta-analysis.' *Applied Psychology: Health and Well-Being.* http://dx.doi.org/10.1111/aphw.12244.

Chapter 14

YIN YOGA FOR SCHIZOPHRENIA

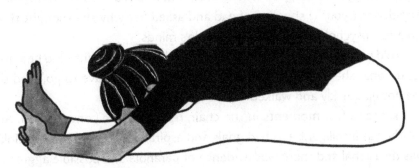

Caterpillar calms the brain, soothes anxiety, and reduces fatigue

I received a referral for testing on a 31-year-old client named Anna who was residing on one of the inpatient units at the hospital. The referral stated that the client was diagnosed with paranoid schizophrenia and was refusing her medications and did not participate in any therapeutic activities.

When I went to meet with Anna the following day, I did not see her in the large day room where many of the clients congregated. I looked in the different smaller rooms, the TV room, game room, and comfort room, but she was not there. When I asked one of the nurses, she shrugged and said, "Probably in her room, she doesn't leave except to eat and use the bathroom." I walked through the darkened hallway into the quiet female dormitory. All the other clients were out, and their doors were open except for the last room on the right. Anna's name was on the door with a handwritten sign that said, "Don't come in." I knocked gently and there was no answer. I knocked again with a little more purpose and I heard a voice, sounding annoyed, say, "What?"

I opened the door slowly and peeked my head in. "Hi Anna, I'm Dr. Meyers. Would it be okay for me to chat with you for a few minutes?" She nodded and I sat down in the chair beside her. She was a pretty woman with dark brown eyes and unkempt hair. She looked younger than her stated age and was dressed in standard-issue gray sweatpants and sweatshirt.

I asked her how she was doing, and she said, "I don't like it here. The staff are jealous of me, especially Maude, the head nurse. She is jealous of my clothes, my mind, and my family." I gently tried to redirect Anna toward her own experiences on the unit, but she continued, "She knows I am the chosen one, God's chosen one. She is going to hell. I will make sure of it."

I asked her about her goals and Anna said, "I am getting married. I already have 16 children and I am going to go home to my husband and my family under the house of God." Anna's voice became animated as she continued to share about her children, her company she owned, and her college degree in psychology. She stopped talking after a moment and said, "You think I'm stupid, don't you?" I shook my head and asked her why she thought this. "I am a real psychologist. I can read people's minds."

I told her that I thought she was very intelligent and wanted to hear more about what she was experiencing. She said, "I can't. I have to go," and then she got up quickly and walked away.

I sat for a few moments in the chair, reviewing the conversation. Anna clearly was intelligent and had goals and aspirations, however, her thinking was delusional and there was evidence of paranoia and possible aggression. I went into the nursing station to read her chart. It was two volumes, which indicated that she had a long mental health history. I sat for the next two hours reading about her life. Anna had been born with fetal alcohol syndrome, exposed to both cocaine and alcohol in utero. She had experienced sexual and physical abuse by her uncle, who was eventually sent to prison. She was removed from the home when she was ten years old and her parents were found not able to care for her. Her mental health issues had started at this time, including suicidal ideation and psychosis, and she had lived in various group homes, residential centers, and psychiatric institutions most of her adolescence and adult life.

Anna had several psychiatric diagnoses, including bipolar disorder, schizo-affective disorder, schizophrenia, PTSD, and cocaine dependence. She had spent time in juvenile detention for assaulting staff in her group home. As an adult, she had been in and out of drug rehabilitation centers, psychiatric hospitals, and supervised apartments with crisis management. She had been on many medications, including antipsychotics. When I met her on the inpatient unit, she had already been there for two months and there were no discharge plans on the horizon.

YIN YOGA FOR SCHIZOPHRENIA

Over the next month, I attempted to complete our standard intellectual and personality testing with Anna, but every time I would attempt to work with her, she would ultimately refuse after spending a few minutes talking and sharing her concerns which were often part of her larger delusion about being "God's chosen one."

It became clear to me that she was not going to tolerate a standard battery of tests. As I was writing a note in her chart indicating that the client was "not testable," I saw Anna out of the corner of my eye in the day room. There was music playing and she was swaying back and forth, making graceful movements with her arms in rhythm to the music. I watched her move and flow with her eyes closed and a soft smile on her face. She looked relaxed and at ease and even carefree.

I went into the dayroom and asked Anna if I could dance with her. She looked at me, shook her head in disbelief, and started to laugh. "Go ahead lady, but I am a ballerina and an all-star." I laughed and said, "I am a terrible dancer, but I love to dance anyway." She gestured for me to accompany her, and we danced and swayed to the music. I added a couple of yoga moves, gently doing some arm circles and Half Sun Salutations. She immediately followed along and gracefully dipped and moved her body. I added in a Standing Warrior, and she imitated me perfectly. Wordlessly, we continued to do this yoga dance, moving through a variety of standing poses. Finally, I went into Tree pose, and she did the same. We fell out at the same time and started laughing in unison. "You're not that bad," she reassured me. We were both a bit breathless and warm. "Want to do this again some time?" I asked her. "Maybe," she said, and walked away.

Over the next few months, I continued to visit with Anna, but left my clipboard behind. I brought my phone and mini speaker and would play different songs that we could dance to. We would move and flow without speaking much, and I watched how Anna would relax and close her eyes and look at ease for several minutes at a time. One day, I asked her if she would like to do yoga with me. She immediately got angry and accused me of wanting her to do the devil's work. "That goes against God."

I immediately reversed course and asked her to just dance with me again, but she was not having it. She refused to meet with me for the next several weeks and her nurse reported that she was becoming more and more withdrawn and would not leave her room. She was refusing her medications. Her doctor decided to try Clozaril, a medication that can be helpful when clients don't respond to at least two different antipsychotics. Over the next two weeks, Anna started to come around and she was more visible on the unit.

She started to smile again at times and even said hello to me, letting me know that she no longer thought I was trying to harm her.

I asked her if she would be willing to do some dancing and movement. I asked her to pick a song she would like, and she chose an upbeat song from the '80s band Tears for Fears, called "Everybody Wants to Rule the World." We moved and danced together.

As the music ended, I asked her if we could just "rest" for a few minutes on the floor. She agreed and I laid out two yoga mats and blankets and we just rested next to each other. She kept her eyes open, and I stayed quiet and focused on breathing fully and completely. Her breathing slowed down, and she began to breathe in rhythm with me. We stayed like that for about ten minutes. At the end, she turned to me and said, "God loves you."

Each week, I would do this simple practice of movement and quiet breathing with Anna. Occasionally, I would stretch and take a yin shape, selecting one of the following: Caterpillar, Half Butterfly, and Dragonfly. Anna would follow along provided I did not talk or make eye contact. Eventually, she was deemed "discharge ready." She had been compliant with her medication and was able to participate in groups. I came to say goodbye to her. She made eye contact with me and said quietly, "You are a terrible dancer." We laughed and I hugged her and wished her well.

Our yoga together had not been traditional. We used a variety of poses, movements, music, breath work, and even some longer yin poses. By letting her mind find space to rest in the quietude, she found peace at times, laughter during the music, and human connection.

Schizophrenia is a chronic and severe mental illness characterized by distortions in thinking, perception, language, sense of self, and behavior. It is considered a psychotic disorder in that the person's perception of reality is impaired with symptoms of hallucinations, delusions, and cognitive impairment. The prevalence of schizophrenia is hard to pinpoint with good accuracy, due to the overlap with other psychotic disorders and the complexity of the diagnosis itself. Therefore, most prevalence estimates typically combine schizophrenia with other psychotic disorders. It is estimated that there are around 20 million people with schizophrenia worldwide. In the US, the prevalence of schizophrenia and other psychotic disorders is less than 1 percent of the population (in the range of 0.25% to 0.64%).[1, 2]

While the prevalence of schizophrenia is much lower than that of mood and anxiety disorders, it has a much greater health, social, and disability impact on those suffering from it. Those with schizophrenia have a morbidity risk two to three times higher than those without and are at increased risk for premature mortality.[3, 4] This is likely due to co-occurring medical conditions, including heart disease, diabetes, and liver disease, which may be due to medication side-effects, as well as the under-detection and under-treatment of underlying medical issues. In addition, about half of individuals who suffer from schizophrenia have co-occurring mental health conditions, including substance use disorders, depression, and anxiety. Due to the severity and chronicity of the symptoms of schizophrenia, there are also higher financial costs associated with this condition as compared to other mental and physical health conditions. In fact, schizophrenia is one of the top 15 leading causes of disability worldwide.[5] The direct and indirect costs associated with schizophrenia include unemployment, criminal justice involvement, social service needs, and medical costs.

Schizophrenia is considered a chronic brain disorder and one of a spectrum of psychotic disorders. Psychosis refers to a loss of reality caused by a disruption in the way the brain processes information. It is a complex diagnosis which is often misunderstood because it has several components. People often confuse schizophrenia with "split personality" or "multiple personalities" or assume a person with schizophrenia is violent or dangerous. This view is reinforced by media reports on violent crimes committed by someone who is mentally ill. In fact, most people with schizophrenia are not dangerous or violent and they are more likely to be the victims rather than the perpetrators of violence.[6] However, there is a subset of people with schizophrenia who can behave violently, especially if there is a substance abuse co-morbidity.[7]

Schizophrenia is considered a heterogenous clinical syndrome with a good deal of variance between individuals suffering from this condition. People with limited mental health resources will often end up homeless, have frequent hospitalizations, or find themselves in prison. But most people living with schizophrenia are able to live with their families, or on their own in a supported living environment.

Schizophrenia is generally divided into three major categories: positive symptoms (delusions, hallucination, paranoia), negative symptoms (the absence or loss of the ability to initiate actions, speak, express feelings, loss of pleasure), and disorganized symptoms (confused thinking and speech, impaired logic, bizarre behaviors, abnormal movements).[8] Positive symptoms describe conditions that relate to psychosis, an indication that there has been loss of contact with reality in which a person's thoughts, perceptions, and beliefs are disturbed in some way that makes it hard for them to distinguish what is real and what is internally created by the mind.[9] The DSM-5 describes schizophrenia and other psychotic disorders both in terms of symptoms and level of severity.[10]

Schizophrenia typically strikes people somewhere in their late teens to mid-thirties, but most commonly occurs in early to mid-twenties for males and mid- to late twenties for females. This often coincides with college or early adulthood, which is particularly heartbreaking for the individuals and their families, as their lives are just beginning. Typically, the earlier the onset, the worse the prognosis, with many variables impacting the overall course of the illness, including premorbid adjustment, educational achievement, and environment. The onset is typically gradual, with a high incidence of depression and impaired or altered cognition prior to the emergence of psychosis.

Adding to the complexity of schizophrenia is the fact that the course and outcome of the disorder are variable and not easily predicted. While most people have a chronic course with frequent exacerbations and remission of symptoms and ongoing progressive deterioration, there are some that have a more positive course of recovery (about 20%), and a small number recover completely from the disorder. It is not clear why this is the case, but it adds to the challenges in treatment, particularly for the majority of clients that struggle with life-long symptoms.[11, 12] Co-occurring psychiatric disorders, including depression (30–54%), PTSD (29%), obsessive-compulsive disorder (23%), and panic disorder (15%), are common and may present additional challenges to those individuals with schizophrenia.[13]

The causes of schizophrenia are multifactorial and include genetic, physio-logical, and environmental factors. There is a strong genetic component with schizophrenia, although researchers are still determining both the complex genetic variations and mutations along with the epigenetics that contribute to the expression of the disease. The risk of schizophrenia is approximately 10 percent for a first-degree relative and 3 percent for a second-degree relative.[14] Studies of identical twins have consistently shown a concordance rate of approx-imately 50 percent (that is, chances of the second twin having schizophrenia if the first twin has been diagnosed is about 50%).[15] The largest twin study to date, looking at data from over 30,000 pairs of twins in Denmark from 1870 to the present, found that as much as 79 percent of the risk for someone to develop schizophrenia may be explained by genetic factors.[16] In other words, genes contribute much more substantially in terms of whether someone develops schizophrenia than previous estimates indicated.

New research has found some genetic overlap of schizophrenia with autism and bipolar disorders.[17] Other factors contributing to schizophrenia may include pregnancy and birth complications, and prenatal and perinatal stress, and even the season of birth has been linked to the incidence of schizophrenia.[18] As more genetic discoveries and neuroscientific advances continue, further understand-ing of the physiology of schizophrenia will facilitate better treatment.

Other disorders on the psychotic spectrum include schizoaffective disorder—which includes both a major mood episode and psychotic symptoms similar to schizophrenia—substance-induced psychotic disorder, psychotic disorder due to a medical condition, and catatonia associated with another mental disorder. For the sake of simplicity, in this chapter I will be focusing primarily on schizophrenia, but many of the treatment interventions, including yoga and meditation, apply to the spectrum of psychotic disorders.

Treatment for schizophrenia has evolved and changed significantly over the centuries. Prior to 1800, people with mental illness were living on the streets, in jails, or in mental "asylums." During the 19th century, wide-scale use of hospitals to treat people with mental health disorders began and led to long periods of institutionalization of many people with schizophrenia and other serious mental health problems.

In 1887, German psychiatrist Emil Kraepelin formally categorized the symptoms of schizophrenia as *dementia praecox* (dementia of early life), believing that this disorder occurred early in life and was similar to senile dementia. In 1911, Swiss psychiatrist Eugen Bleuler first utilized the term *schizophrenia,* which came from the root *schizo* meaning "split" and *phrene* meaning "mind." Bleuler was reflecting the cognitive confusion and disordered thinking that characterize the illness, rather than multiple personality disorder (which is a completely different disorder altogether). Bleuler recognized that schizophrenia was a group of diseases with primary and accessory symptoms (similar to the modern understanding of positive and negative symptoms), and these became the early typology for modern-day categories presented in the DSM-5 and other systems.[19]

For many decades following Kraepelin's and Bleuler's descriptions of schizophrenia, there were very few treatments available, and those were often risky and ineffective. Insulin coma, barbiturate-induced sleep therapy, frontal lobotomies, and leukotomies (cutting the nerve tracts of the frontal lobes to reduce agitation) were utilized with extreme risk to the client, including heart attack, stroke, or cognitive impairment following psychosurgery. By the mid-1950s, thousands of clients were warehoused in large psychiatric hospitals, often for most of their lives, with poor quality of life. A breakthrough came in the 1950s with the first effective antipsychotic drug, chlorpromazine (known by the brand name Thorazine). This medication was found to reduce agitation and mood disturbance along with positive symptoms like delusions and hallucinations and even some of the more intractable negative symptoms. Further, Thorazine shortened hospitalizations and improved overall quality of life.

Continued exploration of psychopharmacology led to a greater understanding of the role of neurotransmitters such as dopamine, serotonin, and glutamate that may be involved in the pathophysiology of schizophrenia. However, medications alone did not provide a cure. Some clients with schizophrenia did not respond to medications or had severe and disabling side-effects. The de-institutionalizing of clients in the 1960s and 1970s led to increased rates of relapse of illness, homelessness, and prison for many people suffering from schizophrenia. It became clear that supportive psychotherapy including social skills, vocational rehabilitation, housing, and case management needed to be integrated into treatment to prevent relapse. In the late 20th century, there were important breakthroughs in neuroimaging, genetic studies, and pharmacological discoveries. These breakthroughs, along with a better understanding of the role of both medication and a psychosocial rehabilitation approach, have improved outcomes in people suffering from schizophrenia.[20, 21]

Even with all the advances in treatment over the last 20 years, there are still many challenges in treating people with schizophrenia. First and foremost, sufferers continue to experience a number of residual symptoms, many falling into the negative symptom category, that can impact their overall quality of life. The research shows that negative symptoms are associated with worse overall functional outcomes even when positive symptoms are well controlled by medications. In addition, medications which are considered the first line of treatment due to their ability to reduce acute symptoms—including positive symptoms such as delusions and hallucinations—often have side-effects, including obesity and dyslipidemia, and either do not treat the negative symptoms or lead to worsening depression, fatigue, poor motivation, and cognitive slowing.

Non-pharmacological interventions, including cognitive behavioral therapy (CBT), vocational rehabilitation, and social skills training, are widely accepted as important adjunctive treatments in addition to medications. However, the research has shown that many of these interventions have not impacted the more chronic and debilitating negative symptoms of schizophrenia. Only CBT and social skills training have shown any promising improvement in negative symptoms, but it is not clear if these modalities alone are effective.[22, 23] The APA reflected this in their guide for clinical treatment of schizophrenia: "There is no treatments with proven efficacy for primary negative symptoms."[24]

Given the lack of effective treatments for the negative symptoms of schizophrenia, coupled with the ongoing challenges of co-morbid medical and psychiatric illnesses, there is a growing interest in integrative and innovative approaches to treating schizophrenia spectrum disorders. These include exercise, cognitive remediation training, and yoga.

Yoga therapy has been explored as an adjunctive treatment for schizophrenia because of the inconsistent and sometimes non-responsiveness to antipsychotic medications especially for the negative symptoms of schizophrenia. In addition, there are side-effects of antipsychotic medications including metabolic syndrome, endocrinological and menstrual dysfunction. However, prior to the last two decades, these studies were limited due to a number of factors, such as accessibility to yoga, poor adherence and high dropout rates, and a feeling that individuals with schizophrenia might not be able to participate in fully in yoga due to physical limitations and inability to follow directions, or that it could even exacerbate psychosis.[25, 26]

More recently, there has been much more promising research supporting the use of yoga for this population, with several controlled studies of it as a viable evidence-based intervention for schizophrenia. Results from these studies have shown evidence of symptom reduction in psychosis and depression.[27, 28] In addition, yoga has been shown to improve negative symptoms associated with schizophrenia, an area where traditional treatment such as medications and psychotherapy have not been highly efficacious. While these studies have been small, there are exciting findings coming out in different inpatient and outpatient settings suggesting the efficacy of yoga as an adjunctive treatment for negative symptoms of schizophrenia.[29, 30, 31] Further, yoga was not reported to have any adverse events or side-effects for this client population, which is significant, given the risks of traditional pharmacological treatments.[32]

Another area of promising research for patients with schizophrenia is the effect of yoga on social cognition. Recent studies have looked at facial emotion recognition deficits which are common challenges for this population.[33, 34, 35] Facial emotion recognition deficits (FERD) have been correlated with impaired social and occupational functioning, as the ability to discriminate facial emotions is an important component in prosocial relationships. In addition, studies have found that oxytocin, an amino acid peptide hormone, plays a role in helping people to accurately perceive positive social cues, which can facilitate interpersonal relationships in terms of closeness and trust.[36] Researchers have found that yoga therapy can improve plasma oxytocin levels in schizophrenia clients which in turn can lead to improved FERD and social functioning, and a reduction in negative symptoms.[37]

The biological underpinnings of yoga therapy for schizophrenia are just beginning to be understood. Yoga researchers Shivarama Varambally, Sanju George, and Bangalore Nanjundaiah Gangadhar have been exploring the different mechanisms of action for yoga and psychiatric disorders such as schizophrenia, and write that "postulated mechanisms of action include: (a) modulation of the hypothalamic-pituitary-adrenal (HPA) axis; (b) enhancement of GABAergic neurotransmission; (c) autonomic modulation; and (d) neuroendocrinological effects."[38]

In addition to oxytocin, other studies that looked at hormones such as cortisol and brain-derived neurotropic factor (BDNF) have found that blood cortisol levels decreased while BDNF levels increased in yoga groups that were experiencing depression, a common co-morbidity with schizophrenia. This is important because sustained higher levels of cortisol that cause lowered levels of BDNF ultimately can lead to grey matter loss and possible cognitive impairment.[39] Preliminary studies have shown that yoga can also be a protective factor against cognitive decline when clients are receiving electroconvulsive therapy (ECT), a treatment option for some individuals with schizophrenia.[40]

Given the complex interplay of genetic and biological factors in the expression of schizophrenia spectrum disorders, it is even more challenging to pinpoint specific mechanisms of action. In addition, yoga research for this client population can be difficult due to the interaction of yoga with psychopharmacology, the challenge of how to measure change in people with complex psychiatric and biological disorders, and the selection of appropriate yoga given the variety of yoga practices that are available.

In India, the National Institute of Mental Health and Neurosciences (NIMHANS) has initiated both the research and practice of yoga for people across the mental health spectrum. B.N. Gangadhar, a researcher, psychiatrist, and pioneer in yoga therapy for mental health, states that "Yoga can be successfully integrated with clinical psychiatry practice."[41] In the United States and other countries, there is a growing movement toward this integration in psychiatry; however, in my clinical experience, there are few yoga programs for clients with serious mental illness, including schizophrenia.

It is important to note that yoga is in no way a substitute for other evidence-based treatment for schizophrenia, including medications to manage psychotic symptoms. The stories that I will share of yoga in inpatient settings for individuals with schizophrenia are part of larger comprehensive treatment plans for each of these clients.

When I started introducing yoga to my inpatient clients, there was a lot of resistance from the treatment teams around trying yoga for those suffering from schizophrenia. While I recognized that yoga is not a substitute for other evidence-based treatment for schizophrenia, including medications to manage psychotic symptoms, I believed that yoga could be part of a larger comprehensive treatment plan for clients. However, the nursing staff felt that our inpatient individuals were "too psychotic" or "too aggressive" to participate. When a yoga class was announced over the building PA system, the clients that were sent to my class were typically the "higher functioning" ones who were close to discharge and were interested in learning new practices for life outside the hospital.

I decided that instead of waiting for the more impaired clients to come to me, I would have to go to them. Never one to shy away from a challenge, I decided to go to the forensic unit of the hospital. The building is foreboding, with its circular shape around a courtyard and tall fences akin to a prison yard. In order to get into the building, I had to pass through a metal detector and speak to state police officers about the purpose of my visit.

Usually, the officers waved me in as I came by with my briefcase or clipboard doing "psychology duties." On that day, one of the officers stopped me as he saw my yoga mat and bolster moving through the detector system. He smirked and said, "Are you visiting yogi bear?" I smiled casually, pretending that this was funny, and said, "Officer Jones, you should come do yoga with me." He laughed and said that he was so inflexible he would never get up off the floor.

We both laughed at this and I moved on through the dank, green hallway toward the locked wards. When I entered the long-term care ward, I was struck by how the clients were all tucked away in their small rooms. There was not much going on in the hallways except for nursing staff with clipboards, housekeeping doing some mopping, and the noise of doors opening and closing.

As I walked by the clients' rooms, some looked at me, but most were reading, sleeping, or staring into space. I heard one client yelling and saw him running around the unit without any clothing on. My heartbeat rapidly accelerated and I felt a strong urge to run away. The staff escorted him back to his room, and I went to find the head nurse and was told he was in the break room, where I then found him, a burly man named Steve in his early forties. I introduced myself and explained that I wanted to do some yoga with any of the clients who might be interested.

He paused for a minute and then said to one of the staff sitting next to him, "Hey, how about Robert?" The other man slowly smiled and said, "Oh, yeah, Robert likes yoga. I'm sure he would be happy to participate. I'll take you to him." The men smiled and nodded at me encouragingly. I felt apprehensive, but pleased that they were able to so quickly find a client for me to work with.

Robert was lying in his small bed. He was a tall man, about 30 years old, long blond hair with a thin frame. "Robert, there's someone here to see you," said the staff. Robert looked up at me curiously. "Hi Robert, I'm Tracey. I'm starting a new program here, using yoga to help with stress and well-being. Would you be interested in doing a short practice with me?"

I heard a few suppressed laughs behind me and saw that a crowd of three or four staff members was now watching.

Robert smiled and said, "Sure, that sounds good."

I rolled out two mats and began demonstrating some gentle stretches and breath work. Robert looked uncomfortable sitting upright, so I gently offered him a bolster and helped him to sit on the edge to find more ease. I heard more laughing, and I looked up to see Steve and two other staff members laughing and poking each other. Robert and I ignored them, and I continued to lead him through some warm-ups and then did a Supported Bridge, once again helping to center the bolster under him. Now, there was audible laughing outside the room, and I could feel myself getting upset, but I continued to lead Robert through Bridge, Reclining Twist, and *Savasana*.

At the end of the session, Robert looked me directly in the eye and said, "Thank you. You are the first person to spend time with me in a long time."

I heard one of the staff outside the room say, "Who would want to spend time with him?" I chose to ignore this and looked Robert directly in the eyes, as I said, "Thank you for participating today, Robert. You did great." I shook his hand and packed up the yoga mats and left.

As I was walking down the hall, a female staff member came up to me and said, "You should never do yoga with Robert. He's crazy. He can attack people out of the blue. That's why he's in here. The guys wanted to scare you because they think that doing anything kind with the clients is coddling them."

I thanked her for telling me this and quickly left the unit, vowing never to come back. I looked up Robert's record when I got back to my office. The female staff member had been truthful: Robert had a long history of violence in the community when he went off his medications. He had been diagnosed with paranoid schizophrenia, bipolar type, and when he was psychotic, he became aggressive and physically assaultive.

He had been at the hospital for more than five years and had been stable over the past years on his treatment regimen of Clozaril, a powerful antipsychotic that can be highly effective in managing psychotic symptoms (the same medication given to Anna while I was working with her). However, Robert's negative symptoms of schizophrenia had increased, including depression, anhedonia (lack of pleasure), and decreased energy. He was spending most of his time in bed with the exception of meals. I tried to reconcile the man I had worked with that morning with the client's chart that was open in front of me. Should I put myself in harm's way only to find that yoga did not help him?

Did I have enough courage to walk back onto the unit, head (and yoga mat) held high, and try to work with Robert again?

The answer was yes, I wanted to try again.

The second time I came to the long-term care unit, I had a new approach. I had made copies of different yoga poses and some basic information about the practice. I asked Steve, the head nurse, if I could speak to him and a few of the staff about yoga. Steve looked bemused, but he agreed to get a few of them into the break room. I heard him say, "Hey, that yoga lady came back again. She wants to make you turn into a pretzel."

A few of the staff came in, including the woman who had warned me about Robert. I asked if any of them had ever done yoga. One said that he loved Bikram yoga (otherwise known as hot yoga). Another said that his wife loved yoga. People started to chat a little about it. I asked them if I could lead them through a short series of standing yoga.

I had them do some three-part breath, alternate nostril breathing, and Mountain with arm circles, just about seven minutes of practice. They were laughing at times during the practice, but something had shifted in the room, from skepticism to—dare I say—a little joy.

When we were done, I asked directly, "Do you think Robert is able to participate in yoga? I would like to work with him again, but I'm scared to go alone into his room because I don't know him." The staff member who did Bikram yoga said, "Yeah, I think he could. I'll go with you and let's see if we can get him to do a little."

As we approached Robert's room, I felt my body relax; I knew there was at least a possibility that yoga could become a part of Robert's treatment. As I walked into his room, I saw a smile on his face as he looked at the yoga mat I was holding. He got up and said, "I'm ready."

Over the next several years, I began teaching yoga to many clients with schizophrenia and other psychotic disorders. I found that the positive symptoms of schizophrenia, including hallucinations or delusions, were not the biggest barrier. In fact, because yoga is a quiet practice that can be done without words, many of my clients seemed just fine with limited dialogue and simply following along by watching me. The biggest barrier was the physical conditioning of the clients. Nearly all my clients were on several medications, including antipsychotics, mood stabilizers, antidepressants, and anxiolytics, along with ones for hypertension, diabetes, cholesterol, and pain. As a result, they were extremely tired, slow in their movements, and had difficulty with coordination. I found that even getting on the floor was too challenging for many of them.

Yin yoga became the perfect vehicle to introduce my clients to yoga. I would lead the practice at the bedside more often than on the floor because of the ease it provided my clients to simply take some shapes without having to worry about dizziness, balance issues, or putting movements together. My favorite sequences utilized bolsters and blankets to help stabilize hips, lower backs, and knees, as we spent time in Reclining Butterfly, Reclining Twist, Figure Four, Supported Bridge, Supported Fish, Side-Lying Position, and variations on these poses. I would gently guide these practices using simple cues and frequent reminders to focus on the breath, and often, I would ask them to verbalize how they were feeling from moment to moment.

Using simple but frequent cueing was helpful for my clients to maintain their focus and not get lost in their thoughts. I would use concrete cues and avoid abstract language that might be confusing like "bring your awareness," instead telling them, "Move your left ankle back and forth." I encouraged them to keep their eyes open and grounded in the senses if they started to drift into their own minds and seemed to disconnect from the present moment.

I might ask, "What do you notice right now?" or "Tell me where you feel the sensations right now." This "right now" language was helpful in keeping them present without directly saying they had to pay attention. I would also offer gentle lovingkindness practices, especially toward the end of the routine, to support the cultivation of more positive emotions such as a sense of well-being and positive self-identity. Lovingkindness meditation practices have been shown to be effective in enhancing positive emotions, although more research needs to be done with various clinical populations.[42] I found that these gentle reminders were very helpful for some of my clients, and I would often follow up with a written sign bearing one or more of these phrases, which they could put on their wall as a reminder. Because these practices were easy to follow, I would often pull in nursing staff to do the practices with the clients, so that they could be done several times a week. As on the forensic unit, I often had to work with the staff first to try to get them to "buy in" to the benefits of yoga before they were open to practicing it with the clients.

I had a group of staff that became very interested in yoga and even enrolled in a yoga teacher training program that was offered in the local community. I began incorporating specific yin sequences as part of the treatment plans, putting in a list of poses and goals utilizing traditional psychiatric language. This helped to create a role for yoga as an integrative modality rather than just a fun leisure activity. The clients liked this as well, as they would get "credit" for participation in treatment and also do something that was different from traditional walking around the courtyard or sitting in a social skills group.

A sample treatment plan might look something like this:

> Treatment: Client x will participate in yin yoga program for 30 minutes, three times per week.
>
> Goal: Improve coping skills to manage stress.
>
> Objective 1: Client will utilize breathing exercises when anxious or upset.
> Objective 2: Client will verbalize one to three positive attributes about themselves.
> Objective 3: Client will express feelings directly to staff using "I feel..."
>
> Goal: Increase adherence to healthy lifestyle activities.
>
> Objective 1: Client will participate in gentle movement and stretching to increase flexibility and strength.
> Objective 2: Client will verbalize at least two benefits of yoga, meditation, and other exercise for their overall well-being.
> Objective 3: Client will practice at least one new pose each week to increase endurance and range of motion.

While there are certainly challenges in working with individuals with serious mental illness like schizophrenia, including physical limitations, lack of initiation, and resistance to trying something new, I found that many of the clients were quite open to trying yoga and appreciated the opportunity to do something new and holistic. With the help of the nursing staff, I learned when to approach clients, and when to put a pause on the yoga if a client was not doing well and was not able to participate due to increased psychosis, aggression, or physical illness. Over time, my hospital ordered yoga mats, bolsters, and blocks for the entire hospital so that every unit could incorporate yoga routines as part of the daily schedule. Treatment plans contained a new section devoted to integrative modalities. Yoga now has a place in prisons, psychiatric hospitals, and day treatment rehabilitation programs and is seen an important component of well-being and quality of life.

ENDNOTES

1   www.nimh.nih.gov/health/statistics/schizophrenia
2   www.who.int/news-room/fact-sheets/detail/schizophrenia
3   www.nimh.nih.gov/health/statistics/schizophrenia
4   McGrath, J., Saha, S., Chant, D., and Welham, J. (2008) 'Schizophrenia: A concise overview of incidence, prevalence, and mortality.' *Epidemiologic Reviews, 30,* 67–76.
5   GBD 2016 Disease and Injury Incidence and Prevalence Collaborators (2017) 'Global, regional, and national incidence, prevalence, and years lived with disability for 328 diseases and injuries for 195 countries, 1990-2016: A systematic analysis for the Global Burden of Disease Study 2016.' *Lancet, 390,* 10100, 1211–1259.
6   Wehring, H.J., and Carpenter, W.T. (2011) 'Violence and schizophrenia.' *Schizophrenia Bulletin, 37,* 5, 877–878.
7   Fazel, S., Gulati, G., Linsell, L., Geddes, J.R., and Grann, M. (2009) 'Schizophrenia and violence: Systematic review and meta-analysis.' *PLoS Medicine, 6,* 8, e1000120.
8   https://www.psychiatry.org/patients-families/schizophrenia/what-is-schizophrenia
9   www.nimh.nih.gov/health/publications/understanding-psychosis
10 American Psychiatric Association (2013) *Diagnostic and Statistical Manual of Mental Disorders* (5th ed.) (DSM-5). Arlington, VA: APA.
11 https://www.psychiatry.org/patients-families/schizophrenia/what-is-schizophrenia
12 www.therecoveryvillage.com/mental-health/schizophrenia/related/schizophrenia-statistics/#gref
13 www.therecoveryvillage.com/mental-health/schizophrenia/related/schizophrenia-statistics/#gref
14 McDonald, C., and Murphy, K.C. (2003) 'The new genetics of schizophrenia.' *Psychiatric Clinics of North America, 26,* 1, 41–63.
15 Cardno, A. (2002) 'Twin studies of schizophrenia: From bow-and-arrow concordances to Star Wars mx and functional genomics.' *American Journal of Medical Genetics, 97,* 1, 12–17.
16 Elsevier (2017) 'Largest twin study pins nearly 80% of schizophrenia risk on heritability.' *Science Daily,* October 5. www.sciencedaily.com/releases/2017/10/171005103313.htm.
17 www.therecoveryvillage.com/mental-health/schizophrenia/related/schizophrenia-statistics/#gref
18 www.therecoveryvillage.com/mental-health/schizophrenia/related/schizophrenia-statistics/#gref
19 Jablensky, A. (2010) 'The diagnostic concept of schizophrenia: Its history, evolution, and future prospects.' *Dialogues in Clinical Neuroscience, 12,* 3, 271–287.
20 Lavretsky, H. (2008) 'History of Schizophrenia as a Psychiatric Disorder.' In Musser, K.T., and Jeste, D.J. (eds) *Clinical Handbook of Schizophrenia.* New York: Guilford Press.
21 Tueth, M.J. (1995) 'Schizophrenia: Emil Kraepelin, Adolph Meyer, and beyond.' *Journal of Emergency Medicine, 13,* 6, 805–809.
22 Wykes, T., Steel, C., Everitt, B., and Tarrier, N. (2008) 'Cognitive behavior therapy for schizophrenia: Effect sizes, clinical models, and methodological rigor.' *Schizophrenia Bulletin, 34,* 523.
23 Elis, O., Caponigro, J., and King, A. (2013) 'Psychosocial treatments for negative symptoms in schizophrenia: Current practices and future directions.' *Clinical Psychology Review, 33,* 8, 914–928.
24 American Psychiatric Association (2004) *Practice Guideline for the Treatment of Clients with Schizophrenia.* Arlington, VA: APA.
25 Bangalore, N.G., and Varambally, S. (2012) 'Yoga therapy for schizophrenia.' *International Journal of Yoga, 5,* 2, 85–91.
26 Varambally, S., George, S., and Gangadhar, B. (2020) 'Yoga for psychiatric disorders: From fad to evidence-based intervention?' *British Journal of Psychiatry, 216,* 291–293.

27 Sathyanarayanan, G., Vengadavaradan, A., and Bharadwaj, B. (2019) 'Role of yoga and mind-fulness in severe mental illnesses: A narrative review.' *International Journal of Yoga, 12,* 3–28.

28 Vancampfort, D., Vansteelandt, K., Scheewe, T., *et al.* (2012) 'Yoga in schizophrenia: A systematic review of randomized controlled trials.' *Acta Psychiatrica Scandinavica, 126,* 12–20.

29 Visceglia, E., and Lewis, S. (2011) 'Yoga therapy as an adjunctive treatment for schizophrenia: A randomized, controlled pilot study.' *Journal of Alternative and Complementary Medicine, 17,* 7, 601–607.

30 Rao, N.P., Ramachandran, P., Jacob, A., *et al.* (2021) 'Add on yoga treatment for negative symptoms of schizophrenia: A multi-centric, randomized controlled trial.' *Schizophrenia Research, 231,* 90–97. Advance online publication. https://doi.org/10.1016/j.schres.2021.03.021.

31 Varambally, S., Gangadhar, B.N., Thirthalli, J., *et al.* (2012) 'Therapeutic efficacy of add-on yogasana intervention in stabilized outpatient schizophrenia: Randomized controlled comparison with exercise and waitlist.' *Indian Journal of Psychiatry, 54,* 3, 227–232.

32 Balasubramaniam, M., Telles, S., and Doraiswamy, P.M. (2013) 'Yoga on our minds: Systematic review of yoga for neuropsychiatric disorders.' *Frontiers in Psychiatry, 3,* 117.

33 Behere, R.V., Arasappa, R., Jagannathan, A., *et al.* (2011) 'Effect of yoga therapy on facial emotion recognition deficits, symptoms and functioning in clients with schizophrenia.' *Acta Psychiatrica Scandinavica, 123,* 2, 147–153.

34 Jayaram, N., Varambally, S., Behere, R.V., *et al.* (2013) 'Effect of yoga therapy on plasma oxytocin and facial emotion recognition deficits in clients of schizophrenia.' *Indian Journal of Psychiatry, 55* (Suppl 3), S409–S413.

35 Domes, G., Heinrichs, M., Michel, A., Berger, C., and Herpertz, S.C. (2007) 'Oxytocin improves "mind-reading" in humans.' *Biological Psychiatry, 61,* 731–733.

36 Jayaram, N., Varambally, S., Behere, R.V., *et al.* (2013) 'Effect of yoga therapy on plasma oxytocin and facial emotion recognition deficits in clients of schizophrenia.' *Indian Journal of Psychiatry, 55* (Suppl 3), S409–S413.

37 Domes, G., Heinrichs, M., Michel, A., Berger, C., and Herpertz, S.C. (2007) 'Oxytocin improves "mind-reading" in humans.' *Biological Psychiatry, 61,* 731–733.

38 Varambally, S., George, S., and Gangadhar, B. (2020) 'Yoga for psychiatric disorders: From fad to evidence-based intervention?' *British Journal of Psychiatry, 216,* 291–293.

39 Hariprasad, V.R., Varambally, S., Shivakumar, V., Kalmady, S.V., Venkatasubramanian, G., and Gangadhar, B.N. (2013) 'Yoga increases the volume of the hippocampus in elderly subjects.' *Indian Journal of Psychiatry, 55* (Suppl 3), S394–S396.

40 Hariprasad, V.R., Varambally, S., Shivakumar, V., Kalmady, S.V., Venkatasubramanian, G., and Gangadhar, B.N. (2013) 'Yoga increases the volume of the hippocampus in elderly subjects.' *Indian Journal of Psychiatry, 55* (Suppl 3), S394–S396.

41 Gangadhar, B.N. (2020) 'Integration of yoga in clinical psychiatric practice.' *Telangana Journal of Psychiatry, 6,* 2, 110–112.

42 Zeng, X., Chiu, C., Wang, R., Oei, T.P., and Leung, F. (2015) 'The effect of lovingkindness meditation on positive emotions: A meta-analytic review.' *Frontiers in Psychology 6,* 1693.

— Part 2 —

YIN YOGA AND MENTAL HEALTH PRACTICES

Chapter 15

POSE DESCRIPTIONS

The following descriptions are attended as a guide for yin yoga students. They are not intended as a substitute for working with a certified yoga instructor or yoga therapist. In addition, I have included some cautions for each pose that individuals should consider before attempting a pose. This list is not exhaustive but can serve as a guide for individuals to develop a practice that is safe for them. For example, medical conditions such as glaucoma, uncontrolled high blood pressure, migraines, and acute and chronic back pain can be impacted by poses that involve forward folds and backbends. It is important to consult with a medical professional prior to beginning any physical practice especially if an individual has one or more of the conditions listed.

Each description includes whether it is predominately a yin or yang pose, instructions for safely getting into the shape, typical variations, some possible benefits, cautions, primary meridians that are influenced by the pose, and primary target areas that the pose stimulates. For additional resources on the practices of yin yoga and descriptions of yin poses, I recommend Sarah Powers' book *Insight Yoga*, Paul Grilley's book *Yin Yoga Principles and Practices*, Bernie Clark's book *The Complete Guide to Yin Yoga*, and Biff Mithoefer's book *The Yin Yoga Kit*.

BANANA-ASANA (RECLINING SIDE BEND) (YIN)

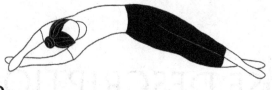

WHAT TO DO

- Begin by lying on back with feet together and arms overhead in one long line
- Clasp hands together or grab opposite elbows
- Keep lower back and buttocks firmly rooted on the floor and begin to move feet and upper body to the right (in the same direction)
- Arch into a crescent (think Standing Half-Moon) or banana shape, elongating left side of body
- Try not to twist or roll onto outer right hip
- As body begins to open more, find appropriate sensations by moving both feet further to right; upper body should also pull in the same direction
- Repeat on other side

PROPS

- Folded blanket or bolster (for shoulder/hands)

VARIATIONS

- To increase sensation, when feet are as far to the side as possible, cross ankles. Likely the greatest stretch will be achieved by crossing outside ankle over inner ankle but crossing the other way might work best for some
- To decrease upper body range of motion, rest arms across chest and simply stretch lower body in crescent shape

BENEFITS

- Great whole side body stretch
- Stretches spine in lateral flexion
- Stretches obliques and intercostal muscles between ribs

CAUTIONS

- Lower back issues

MERIDIANS

- Liver/Gallbladder
- Heart/Lung (if arms are raised overhead)
- Small Intestine/Large Intestine

TARGET AREAS

- Spinal flexion from iliotibial (IT) band to top of rib cage

BREATH OF JOY (PRANAYAMA/YANG)

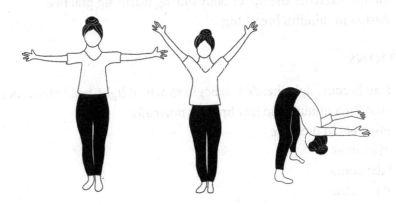

WHAT TO DO

- Stand with feet shoulder-width apart (4–6 inches) and parallel, with knees soft or slightly bent
- Inhale to about one-third of lung capacity and swing arms up in front of body, bringing them parallel to each other at shoulder level (sleep-walker arms) with palms facing ceiling
- Inhale again, filling to two-thirds capacity, and stretch arms out to the side like bird wings at shoulder level
- Inhale to full capacity and swing arms over head, arms parallel, with palms facing each other
- Exhale with an audible sigh or "ha" sound, bending the knees to an appropriate depth toward a standing squat, and swing arms down and behind, like diving into a pool
- Repeat up to 5–10 times, being careful to not strain; avoid becoming light-headed

VARIATIONS

- Inhale and raise arms over head, placing hands on top of upper back
- Exhale with audible sigh, bending the knees toward a standing squat
- Can be done in a chair or seated on the floor

BENEFITS

- Increases oxygen levels in the bloodstream by encouraging deep breathing and full use of lungs
- Increases energy by temporarily stimulating the sympathetic nervous system
- Gently stretches the upper body during warm-up practice
- Assists in mindful breathing

CAUTIONS

- Can become light-headed so begin slowly; if light-headedness occurs, stop for a minute and just breathe normally
- High blood pressure
- Migraines
- Glaucoma
- Back issues

MERIDIANS

- Heart/Lung/Small Intestine/Large Intestine
- Kidney/UB

TARGET AREAS

- Erector muscles (spine)
- Shoulders/arms

BRIDGE/SUPPORTED BRIDGE (YANG/YIN)

WHAT TO DO

- Begin by lying on back with bent knees
- Place feet hip-width apart with knees over ankles, feet parallel

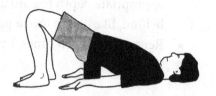

- Flatten shoulders and place hands palm down on floor
- Lengthen neck and as you inhale, press firmly into both feet, lifting pelvis toward ceiling
- *Option:* Keep arms by sides with palms down, or clasp hands underneath buttocks, drawing shoulder blades together
- Engage legs and buttocks to lift hips higher, keeping chin tucked into throat with head on floor
- To release pose, on an exhale, release hands and gently roll spine back down to mat

PROPS

- Block/bolster under hips
- Blanket to support shoulders

VARIATIONS

- Supported Bridge (sometimes called Pontoon): Place block or soft bolster under pelvis to support weight
  - Once pelvis is supported by appropriate prop, walk feet away, straightening legs for deeper intensity
  - This version is more predominately a yin shape and can also be an alternative to other spine extension poses that may not be accessible, including Saddle or Cat Tail
- Breathing Bridge can be done by inhaling and lifting the pelvis toward the ceiling while simultaneously raising arms up and lowering them on the floor behind the head. Exhale and bring arms back up and lower by your sides as your lower pelvis to the floor

BENEFITS

- Strengthens front of thighs (including quadriceps), back muscles, back of thighs (including hamstrings and glutes), and shins
- Stretches chest (including pectoral muscles), front of hips (hip flexors), abdominals, and chest
- Improves posture
- May reduce lower back pain

CAUTIONS

- Back injury
- Arthritic hips/hip replacements

- Eye conditions
- Gastroesophageal reflux disease (GERD); avoid the head below the heart
- Herniated cervical discs
- Neck injuries
- Heart conditions
- High blood pressure
- Low blood pressure
- Neck injury
- Spondylolisthesis
- Shoulder injury
- Pregnancy
- Stroke or cervical artery dysfunction

MERIDIANS

- Spleen/Stomach
- Kidney/UB

TARGET AREAS

- Sacrum/low back (extension)
- Abdominals
- Hip flexors/quadriceps

BUTTERFLY/BOUND ANGLE (YIN)

WHAT TO DO

- From a seated position with legs out-stretched, balance weight equally on both sitting bones (can sit on blanket to elevate hips)
- Bend knees and slide soles of the feet together
- Move feet slightly away from body so legs form a diamond shape
- Allow knees to drop out to each side

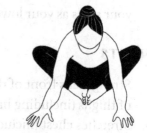

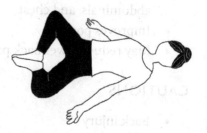

- Bend forward from hips, finding an appropriate stretch in hips, groin, and lower back
- Let the chin to rest down toward the chest, allowing the back to gently round as the body folds forward
- Rest hands lightly on floor or on feet; avoid pulling deeper into the pose

PROPS

- Blanket or cushion to ease hip pain
- Supports under knees or thighs if knees are sensitive or groin is tight
- Bolster (stay upright and place bolster in front of torso for support)

VARIATIONS: RECLINING BUTTERFLY/ RECLINING BOUND ANGLE

- Start in a lying-down position, place the soles of the feet together and slide them away from the body, allowing knees to relax toward the floor
- Place hands lightly on belly, floor, or heart

PROPS

- Rest back on bolster or lie back and rest head on blanket
- Supports under knees or thighs if tight groin or sensitive knees

VARIATIONS: HALF BUTTERFLY

- From a seated position with legs outstretched, balance weight equally on both sitting bones (can sit on blanket to elevate hips)
- Keeping one leg outstretched, bend the other leg and place sole of the foot against inner groin of outstretched leg just above knee
- Allow knee to drop out to one side and keep outstretched leg straight
- Bend forward from hips, finding an appropriate stretch in hips, groin, and lower back
- Let the chin rest toward the chest, allowing the back to gently round as the body folds forward
- Rest the hands lightly on floor or feet and avoid pulling deeper into pose

PROPS

- Blanket or cushion to ease hip pain
- Supports under bent knees or thighs if sensitive or groin is tight
- Support under knee of outstretched straight leg if hamstrings are tight
- Bolster if remaining upright in front of torso for support

BENEFITS

- Stretches muscles supporting the spine
- Stretches the inner thighs (adductors)
- Stretches lower back

CAUTIONS

- Inguinal hernia
- Osteoporosis—caution or avoid rounding forward
- Spinal disc issues

MERIDIANS

- Kidney/UB
- Liver/Gallbladder

TARGET AREAS

- Adductors
- Spinal flexion
- Hamstrings (Half Butterfly)

CAT PULL (YIN)

WHAT TO DO

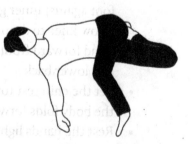

- Start by lying on right side
- Recline head onto right elbow or rest elbow
  on floor and support head in right hand
- Keep bottom (right) leg straight
- Bring top (left) leg forward and to the side
  on a diagonal
- Bend bottom leg and bring heel toward buttock

- Reach back with top (left) hand and grab bottom right foot (using strap around foot if needed)
- Repeat on opposite side

PROPS

- Strap to reach the bottom leg and pull toward buttocks
- Blanket under head/shoulders for comfort and support

VARIATIONS

To decrease intensity:

- Stay propped up on elbow and do not recline head
- Remain supported by right elbow
- Release left hand and maintain bent right knee without holding foot

To increase intensity (yang version):

- Recline head and left shoulder toward floor, looking over left shoulder to bottom foot
- Utilize left hand to pull foot away from buttock

BENEFITS

- Mild compression in low back
- Opens quads/upper thighs
- Counterpose to strong forward bends
- Twist in yang version

CAUTIONS

- Low back issues
- Tight quadriceps

MERIDIANS

- Spleen/Stomach
- Kidney/UB (if back is arched/twisted)

TARGET AREAS

- Spinal extension
- Lumbar/sacrum/rib cage (in twist)

CAT/COW (YANG)

CAT

WHAT TO DO

- Begin in Tabletop (all fours) by placing hands beneath shoulders, knees beneath hips
- On an exhale, press evenly into hands, drawing navel toward spine
- Drop chin to chest as you tuck tailbone under while rounding spine to ceiling
- To release pose, relax abdominals, reversing tilt of hips to come back to neutral Tabletop, or taking counter-pose of Cow

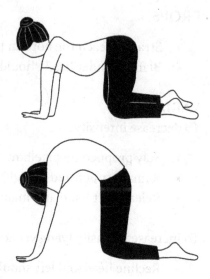

PROPS

- Folded blanket under knees
- Blocks for forearms if wrist/hand pain

VARIATIONS

- Keep neck neutral if neck pain
- For wrist or hand pain can perform on forearms on the floor or on blocks

BENEFITS

- Strengthens upper body (arms, shoulders, chest, abdominals)
- Stretches back and spine, shoulders, front of wrists
- Gentle warm-up for yin/yang practice

CAUTIONS

- Carpal tunnel syndrome
- Spinal disc issues
- Vertigo/dizziness
- Wrist injuries/arthritis in hands/fingers

MERIDIANS

- Kidney/UB
- Spleen/Stomach

TARGET AREAS

- Spinal flexion
- Abdominals

COW

WHAT TO DO

- Begin in Tabletop, with hands beneath shoulders, fingers spread fully, and hips right above knees
- Inhale, lift head slightly, careful not to crunch or strain back of neck, and take gaze up toward ceiling
- Simultaneously, reach tailbone up and toward ceiling, letting spine arch, dropping belly toward the floor
- Exhale, coming back to a neutral Tabletop position, or taking counter-pose of Cat

PROPS

- Folded blanket under knees
- Blocks for forearms if wrist/hand pain

VARIATIONS

- Keep neck neutral if neck pain
- For wrist or hand pain, can perform on forearms on the floor or on blocks

BENEFITS

- Strengthens back, muscles along spine, shoulders, back of wrists, back of neck
- Stretches abdominals, front of wrists, front of neck
- Gentle warm-up for yin/yang practice

CAUTIONS

- Back injury
- Hernia
- Hip injury
- Spondylolisthesis
- Wrist injury/carpal tunnel

MERIDIANS

- Kidney/UB
- Spleen/Stomach

TARGET AREAS

- Spinal extension
- Hips/Abdominals

CATERPILLAR (SEATED FORWARD FOLD) (YIN)

WHAT TO DO

- Begin in seated position (can sit on cushion or blanket), legs outstretched
- Bring chin toward chest and fold forward allowing spine to gently round
- Relax legs and feet

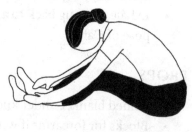
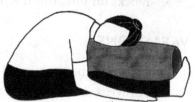

PROPS

- Blankets/cushions beneath sitting bones and/or knees
- Bolster for head/chest

VARIATIONS

- If hamstrings are tight, bend knees and place bolster or blanket underneath; allow back to round fully

- Sit on more cushions/blankets to elevate hips to make it easier to fold forward
- If knees feel strained, activate quadriceps by flexing feet or keep small bend in knees
- If neck feels strained in Caterpillar, support head in hands or rest head on block/bolster
- For deeper relaxation, rest chest on bolster as you round forward (you will not round as deeply in this variation)
- Legs Up the Wall

BENEFITS

- Stresses ligaments along back of the spine
- Compresses stomach in Caterpillar which can help aid digestion
- Produces sense of relaxation with heart below the spine (parasympathetic nervous system response)

CAUTIONS

- Can aggravate sciatica
- Lower back disorders that do not allow for flexion of the spine
- Very tight hamstrings
- Hypermobility can lead to overstretching of lower back and hamstrings

MERIDIANS

- Kidney/UB

TARGET AREAS

- Spinal flexion
- Hamstrings

CHILD (YIN)

WHAT TO DO

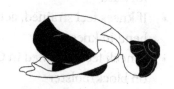

- Begin by coming into Tabletop and lower hips down to heels
- Slowly fold forward by bringing chest toward thighs
- Allow forehead to move toward ground (touch the ground or use block/bolster)

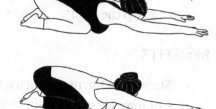

- Allow arms to rest by sides, palms facing down
- If it is comfortable, turn head to one side

PROPS

- Blanket under hips (for tight ankles) and under knees (for knee sensitivity)
- Bolster between knees to support torso to lessen intensity
- Block for head (to support neck)

VARIATIONS

- Preparation for Frog: Bring the knees mat-width apart while continuing to sit on heels
- Stretch arms forward to reduce neck pressure
- Wide-Knee Child for more comfort in the hips (helpful for pregnancy or breathing issues or just to have more space/ease): Spread knees wide apart with feet together to remove pressure from abdomen
- Wide-Knee Child with Twist: Keeping knees wide apart, keeping the toes aimed toward one another, fold chest forward and incline forehead toward floor; reach right arm underneath torso, palm facing up; left arm can remain outstretched or bent around back toward right hip for deeper twist. Repeat on other side

BENEFITS

- Stretches ankles, back, muscles along spine, buttocks (including the gluteal), shins, shoulders

- Can be a gentle counterpose for many backbends
- Turning inward offers comfort when feeling of vulnerability and fear arise
- Easy compression of abdomen stimulates/benefits digestion
- Helpful resting pose when break is needed

CAUTIONS

- Knee concerns may require support or variation
- Ankles/feet may also require padding or support
- Eye conditions
- Active GERD
- Pregnancy
- Vertigo or any tendency to dizziness

MERIDIANS

- Kidney/UB
- Liver/Gallbladder
- Spleen/Stomach (Wide-Knee twist version)
- Heart/Large Intestine (Wide-Knee twist version)

TARGET AREAS

- Spine extension
- Adductors/groin (Wide-Knee version)
- Shoulders (Wide-Knee twist version)

DANGLE/STANDING FORWARD FOLD (YIN/YANG)

WHAT TO DO

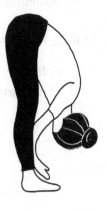

- Begin in Mountain pose with feet hip-width apart, arms by sides
- Gently bend knees and fold forward, bringing head down toward floor (finding appropriate depth for your body)
- Clasp opposite elbows or rest hands on floor

PROPS

- Rest elbows against chair or table to prevent back strain
- Blocks to rest hands in Forward Fold

VARIATIONS

- To decrease intensity in lower back, bend knees more deeply
- For lower back sensitivity, rest elbows against table/chair or on thighs
- To increase intensity: Straighten legs; wrap arms around legs, holding opposite wrists

BENEFITS

- Spinal flexion (for lower spine)
- Stretches hamstrings/quadriceps
- Compresses stomach/internal organs to aid in digestion

CAUTIONS

- High blood pressure
- Glaucoma
- Low blood pressure (when coming out of pose, make sure to stand slowly)
- Back issues (use variations including bending knees, or avoid altogether and assume Caterpillar or Legs Up the Wall)

MERIDIANS

- Kidney/UB
- Liver/Gallbladder
- Spleen/Stomach

TARGET AREAS

- Spinal flexion
- Hamstrings

DEER (YIN)

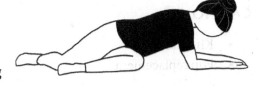

WHAT TO DO

- Start from Sitting Butterfly on floor or Sleeping Swan
- If starting in Butterfly, swing right leg behind you, bringing right heel to buttocks
- Move front (left) leg away from body by advancing left foot (parallel to top of mat) using right angle at left knee as starting point. Right leg can draw up or stretch back relative to body openness
- Remember to keep both sitting bones on the floor
- Sit upright, tilt forward or fold over left leg
- Adjust left knee position for comfort to find appropriate sensation for body
- If starting in Sleeping Swan with right leg outstretched behind, roll all the way on left hip, and bend back right leg to appropriate level of sensation, bringing right heel toward buttocks. Left leg remains in original shape (toward a 90-degree angle)
- Repeat on the opposite side

PROPS

- Support forward knee with blanket
- Support front hip with blanket
- Use bolster to support upper body/torso

VARIATIONS

- To maintain weight equally underneath both hips, move feet more inward toward trunk of body
- To increase sensation, move feet away from both front and back hips/legs
- Twist to stretch side of body by staying upright and twisting front torso toward back foot, looking over opposite shoulder
- Use bolster to support torso and fold forward in a Prone Deer variation

BENEFITS

- Safe and gentle variation of Sleeping Swan

- Balanced internal and external rotation of hip
- Spinal flexion in forward fold version

CAUTIONS

- Knee issues
- Hip replacement

MERIDIANS

- Liver/Gallbladder
- Kidney/UB
- Spleen/Stomach

TARGET AREAS

- Iliotibial (IT) band
- Hip flexors
- Spinal flexion

DOWN DOG (YANG)

WHAT TO DO

- From Tabletop, place hands on mat in front of you, fingers spread wide
- Exhaling, tuck in toes and press evenly into hands and feet while lifting hips toward ceiling (upside down triangle shape)
- Maintaining a long spine, extend heels toward floor (they may not reach all the way to the floor which is perfectly okay). Try extending one heel at a time to open hamstrings. Knees can have a slight bend if hamstrings are tight.
- Check to ensure hands and feet are hip-width apart with even distribution of weight
- Relax neck and let head hang freely as you gaze between feet
- Hold for 30–60 seconds or as long as comfortable

- To release pose, exhale and lower knees to mat, returning to Child's pose

PROPS

- Can use a wedge under palms to reduce pressure on the wrists
- Elevate hands on a block, seat of a chair, or wall to decrease pressure on the shoulders/wrists

VARIATIONS

- Keep knees bent slightly if back is rounded and/or hamstrings are tight
- Separate feet wider on the mat if tight hamstrings prevent heels from reaching the floor
- Can use wall or chair if difficult to get on the floor or if shoulders/wrists are sensitive
- Can place weight on forearms rather than wrists (Dolphin)
- Can do Legs Up the Wall as an alternative to Down Dog to avoid placing weight on hands or wrists

BENEFITS

- Strengthens front of hips (hip flexors), front of thighs (quadriceps), shins, arms, shoulders, upper back
- Stretches back (particularly latissimus dorsi, back of thighs (including gluteals and hamstrings)), arms, calves, front of wrists, and feet

CAUTIONS

- Ear infections
- Eye conditions such as glaucoma
- GERD (may want to avoid head below heart)
- Hernia
- High blood pressure
- Pregnancy: Only stay for short periods of time during 2nd and 3rd trimester
- Vertigo or any tendency to dizziness (e.g., from medications or poorly regulated or unregulated high blood pressure or low blood pressure)

MERIDIANS

- Kidney/UB
- Spleen/Stomach
- Lung/Heart/Small Intestine/Large Intestine

TARGET AREAS

- Spinal flexion
- Shoulder movements
- Hip flexor muscles
- Hamstrings/quadriceps

DRAGONFLY (YIN)

WHAT TO DO

- Start in seated position with legs outstretched at a wide angle
- Widen legs further (finding appropriate level of sensation)
- Sit on a cushion or blanket if needed to tilt hips forward
- Fold forward, placing hands on floor in front or rest elbows on block/bolster

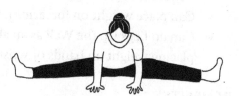
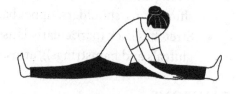
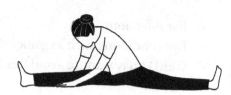

PROPS

- Use a folded blanket/cushion/bolster to raise hips
- Rest elbows on bolster
- Rest chin/forehead on block or bolster
- Place bolster under thighs for tight hamstrings
- Use strap around each foot with knees bent for tight hamstrings

VARIATIONS

- If hamstrings, back, or adductors are tight, bend knees by placing feet flat on floor and bend forward to appropriate level
- For more sensation, move legs toward full split if flexibility permits (careful not to overstretch hamstrings)
- Fold right down onto stomach if appropriate range of motion permits
- Come into Dragonfly Twist by folding over one leg and rotating chest skyward (if flexibility permits, can hold outstretched foot with one or both hands)
- Come into Seated Dragonfly Twist by bringing left hand to outer right thigh and place right fingertips on the mat behind you. Twist from the base of spine to the right (repeat on opposite side)

VARIATIONS: HALF DRAGONFLY

- From a seated position with legs outstretched, balance weight equally on both sitting bones (can sit on blanket to elevate hips)
- Keeping one leg outstretched at a wide angle, bend the other leg and place sole of the foot against inner groin of outstretched leg just above knee
- Allow knee to drop out to one side and keep outstretched leg straight
- Bend forward from hips, finding an appropriate stretch in hips, groin, and lower back
- Let the chin rest toward the chest, allowing the back to gently round as the body folds forward
- Rest the hands lightly on floor or feet and avoid pulling deeper into pose

BENEFITS

- Stretches calves, hamstrings, and adductors (inner thighs)
- Strengthens the quadriceps and spinal muscles
- Opens shoulders/scapula in twist version

CAUTIONS

- Sciatica
- Back issues
- Tight hamstrings (may require a prop)

MERIDIANS

- Kidney/UB
- Liver/Gallbladder
- Spleen/Stomach
- Heart/Lung/Small Intestine/Large Intestine (if twist version)

TARGET AREAS

- Spinal flexion
- Adductors
- Hamstrings
- Obliques/diaphragm (twist version)

DRAGON (YIN)

WHAT TO DO

- Start in Tabletop or in Down Dog
- Step one foot forward between hands
- Forward knee should be right above heel (at 90-degree bend)
- Stretch back leg out
- Adjust as needed to avoid placing full weight on back knee (can use padding under knee if discomfort persists)
- Keep hands on either side of front foot
- Repeat on other side

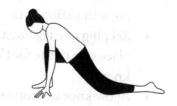
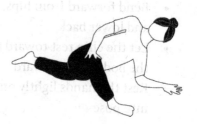

PROPS

- Blanket for back knee if sensitive
- Bolster or blanket to raise back knee if ankle is uncomfortable tucked under
- Blocks for arms to raise trunk off ground

VARIATIONS

There are many variations in Dragon that can be explored. The following are a few of the main alternatives to traditional Dragon:

- For less sensation: Rest arms or hands on front thigh instead of bending forward. Lift chest to increase weight over hips
- For more sensation: Place both hands inside front foot and walk hands forward; lower hips; if range of motion permits, come down on elbows (or rest arms on bolster/block). You can also begin to move into a Dragon Split by straightening both legs into splits and supporting hips with a bolster under buttocks
- To add a twist: Place one hand on front knee and direct it toward the side while the chest rotates toward ceiling
- To deepen hip opener: Roll on outside edge of front foot (pinky toe side) and stay there with knee remaining low to ground; if range of motion permits, come down on elbows or rest them on bolster/block

BENEFITS

- Deep hip and groin opener
- Stretches back leg's hip flexors and quadriceps
- Many variations allow for different sensations in hips/quads

CAUTIONS

- Can be painful for kneecap or tight ankles due to pressure against floor (use blankets/bolster or take variation where torso is upright for less pressure on back leg)

MERIDIANS

- Spleen/Stomach
- Liver/Gallbladder
- Kidney/UB

TARGET AREAS

- Quadriceps
- Hip flexors
- Adductors
- Ankles

FIGURE FOUR

WHAT TO DO

- Start on the back with knees bent and feet on floor
- Place left ankle on top of right knee, creating a "4" shape with left leg
- Thread left arm through opening created, clasping hands behind right thigh, or in front of right shin
- Sacrum rests down to floor as do head and shoulders
- Repeat on opposite side

PROPS

- Strap can be used if too difficult to bring arms around thigh
- Blanket under head or lower back

VARIATIONS

- To decrease sensation, simply cross one ankle on top in Figure Four shape and do not reach for thigh
- If ankles and knees are sensitive, can flex foot that is bent in "4" shape
- If holding knee is not possible, use a strap or the wall, placing left foot on wall with knee bent; sliding closer to wall intensifies stretch

BENEFITS

- Stretches back of thighs (hamstrings)
- Stretches buttocks (including gluteal muscles and piriformis)
- Stretches lower back
- Excellent option for people with knee issues in some other poses (Sleeping Swan)

CAUTIONS

- Hip injury
- Knee injury

MERIDIANS

- Liver/Gallbladder
- Kidney/UB

TARGET AREAS

- Gluteal/piriformis muscle
- Lower back

FISH (YIN)

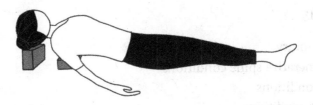

WHAT TO DO

- Begin by lying on back, legs extended, arms resting alongside body, palms down
- Press into forearms and elbows to lift chest, creating arch in upper back that lifts shoulder blades and upper torso from floor
- Keep thighs active and energized, pressing outward through heels as you tilt head back to bring crown of head to floor
- To release pose, press firmly through forearms to slightly lift head off floor. Exhale slowly, lowering torso and then head back to floor

PROPS

- To decrease intensity for head and neck, use two blocks, one directly under shoulders (low-level) and block to support head (mid-level)

VARIATIONS

- To avoid pressure on neck, recline on bolster or thickly rolled blanket, allowing hips to rest on floor and back of head to rest comfortably on support. Arms can release to floor
- Take legs into Butterfly to increase sensation in groin/adductors

BENEFITS

- Improves kyphosis (rounded upper back)
- Improves posture
- Strengthens muscles of back, back of neck, arms, front of the hips (hip flexors), front of thighs (quadriceps), arms, and shoulders
- Stretches shoulders, arms, front of neck, abdominals, and chest

CAUTIONS

- Back injury
- Degenerative spine conditions
- Eye conditions
- Heart conditions
- Hernia
- Herniated cervical discs
- High blood pressure
- Hyperthyroid
- Migraine
- Neck injury
- Osteoarthritis or any joint disease in the neck
- Shoulder injury
- Spinal arthritis or spinal stenosis
- Stroke or cervical artery dysfunction

MERIDIANS

- Spleen/Stomach
- Kidney/UB
- Heart/Lung/Small Intestine/Large Intestine

TARGET AREAS

- Spinal extension
- Abdominal/hip flexor muscles

FIVE-POINTED STAR (YANG)

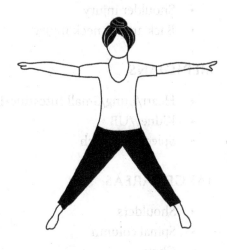

WHAT TO DO

- Begin by standing in Mountain pose
- Step feet wide apart (but still able to maintain balance), pointing forward and parallel to each other
- Press into all four corners of the feet (balls, toes, outer and inner edges); engage quadriceps and glutes by pulling up kneecaps and hugging inner thighs toward each other
- Tuck tailbone down and pull navel into spine to maintain strong core
- Inhale, reaching arms out to sides; lift crown of head toward ceiling and open chest toward front of room
- Exhale, keeping arms up and press into feet, fingers, and crown of head, feeling body expand in five directions
- Do 3–5 rounds and return to Mountain pose

PROPS

- Chair (for seated version)

VARIATIONS

- If shoulder issues are present, bend elbows or place hands on hips
- Seated practice using chair and just arm portion of pose
- To increase sensation, bring arms out wide overhead and take gaze up toward ceiling

BENEFITS

- Improves circulation and respiration
- Stretches spine and chest
- Activates core
- Engages quadriceps and glutes

CAUTIONS

- Shoulder injury
- Back and/or neck injury

MERIDIANS

- Heart/Lung/Small Intestine/Large Intestine
- Kidney/UB
- Spleen/Stomach

TARGET AREAS

- Shoulders
- Spinal column
- Chest

FROG (YIN)

WHAT TO DO

- Begin in Tabletop, with hands beneath shoulders, fingers spread fully, and hips right above knees
- Lower forearms to mat and allow knees to move out to sides of mat, as wide as comfortable
- Allow feet to turn out as you press hips toward back of room, creating a deep stretch in hips and inner thighs
- Three options to moderate intensity:
  - Bring hips more forward if sensations are too intense in groin/hips
  - Keep toes together rather than turn feet out
  - Place hands on floor and keep arms straight by pressing into floor
- Keep gaze between hands, neck neutral

PROPS

- Bolster to rest chest and relax upper body
- Blanket under knees and/or elbows
- Bolster or block under head to support neck

VARIATIONS

- To decrease intensity in groin/hips, start in Child's pose and slide both hands forward, separate knees, but remain sitting on heels (Tadpole pose)
- Another option to decrease intensity is to start by coming into Tadpole pose, then lift hips higher until they are in line with knees, keeping feet together (Half Frog pose)
- To increase intensity, walk hands forward and lower chest to the floor, placing forehead or chin to the ground if flexibility permits

BENEFITS

- Stretches the adductors, hamstrings, and shoulders
- Gentle backbend (spinal extension)

CAUTIONS

- Knees (try using padding)
- Back issues
- Neck stiffness
- Tingling in hands
- Shoulder injury

MERIDIANS

- Spleen/Stomach
- Liver/Gallbladder
- Kidney/UB
- Heart/Lung/Small Intestine/Large Intestine

TARGET AREAS

- Adductors
- Hips (internal rotation)
- Hamstrings
- Shoulders

GODDESS (YANG)

WHAT TO DO

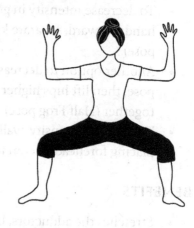

- Begin standing with feet a comfortable distance apart in a wide-leg stance, both feet turned out to about 45 degrees, depending on comfort and ease
- Inhale and extend both arms to shoulder height, while keeping shoulder blades down, then bend elbows so fingertips point up and palms face forward or toward each other
- Exhale, bending knees at the same time so they are directly over ankles
- Make sure shoulder blades remain down and back
- To release pose, inhale and straighten legs while reaching both arms up. Then exhale and release hands, returning to wide-leg stance

PROPS

- Can use chair for seated version

VARIATIONS

- For less shoulder intensity, bring hands together at heart, keeping sensation focus primarily in legs
- For less knee intensity, do not bend knees as deeply
- For more intensity, bring a deeper bend into both knees
- Use chair to decrease intensity for knees by sitting forward in chair, bringing feet out to around 45 degrees, and creating upper body shape, extending arms and bending elbows so palms face forward

BENEFITS

- Strengthens thighs, calves, shoulders, arms, core (including muscles supporting spine and abdominals)
- Stretches muscles of inner thighs (adductors), chest

CAUTIONS

- Hip injury
- Knee injury
- Shoulder injury

MERIDIANS

- Spleen/Stomach
- Liver/Gallbladder
- Heart/Lung/Small Intestine/Large Intestine

TARGET AREAS

- Quadriceps
- Abdominal muscles that support back
- Adductors
- Chest

STIRRUP (HAPPY BABY) (YIN)

WHAT TO DO

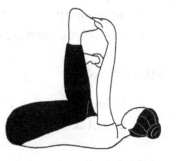

- Begin by lying on back
- Draw knees into chest
- Place a hand on each knee allowing knees to fall as far apart as comfortable
- Slide hands along inside of lower leg to rest, gently weighting leg at shin/ankle
- Catch edges of feet, ankles, or back of calves with hands
- Lift lower legs upright, feet and knees wide apart
- Pull feet down toward floor, finding appropriate level of sensation while keeping tailbone on floor
- Relax head and shoulders down to floor

PROPS

- Folded blanket to support the head
- Strap around soles of feet

VARIATIONS

- To decrease intensity:
  - Take a Half Happy Baby, holding one foot up at a time and keeping other knee hugged into chest
  - Remain at first stage, keeping knees lowered, legs apart, feet turned out, or bring toes together and leave them near groin
- If hamstrings or hips are tight, use belt or strap around soles of feet or brace against a wall
- To increase intensity in hamstrings and hips, gradually straighten legs while pulling feet down

BENEFITS

- Stretches adductors, hamstrings, calves, and low back
- Using arms helps to strengthen biceps
- Releases sacroiliac joints
- Compression of stomach/digestion organs

CAUTIONS

- Hip injury
- Knee injury
- High blood pressure (pose is a mild inversion)

MERIDIANS

- Kidney/UB
- Liver/Gallbladder

TARGET AREAS

- Adductors
- Lumbar spine
- Hips

KNEES INTO CHEST (YIN)

WHAT TO DO

- Begin lying down with legs outstretched
- Bend right knee and interlock fingers below knee
- Keep left leg extended on mat or floor, or bend knee with foot on floor in front of buttocks
- Bring knee in toward chest and hold for at least five breaths
- Release right knee and allow right leg to return to floor
- Repeat with left knee into chest
- Release left knee and allow left leg to return to floor
- *Option:*
  - Hug both knees into chest and hold for several breaths
  - Slowly release both knees and allow legs to float down to floor

PROPS

- Blanket for head and shoulders
- Blanket or folded mat under extended leg to keep it stable

VARIATIONS

- To decrease intensity, make sure to keep opposite foot on floor (with knee bent) rather than straightening leg onto floor
- Bring gentle movement into pose by drawing knee toward armpit and then away from body, opening hip in preparation for Reclining Twist
- To increase intensity, lift head, neck, and shoulders off mat to engage core and bring nose toward knee(s)

BENEFITS

- Strengthens lower back muscles
- Stretches upper back and spine
- Compresses abdomen and pelvic muscles to aid with gas/bloating

CAUTIONS

- High blood pressure

- Neck and back pain (keep shoulders and head on ground)
- Slipped disc and sciatica
- Advanced stages of pregnancy

MERIDIANS

- Kidney/UB
- Spleen/Stomach
- Heart/Lung/Small Intestine/Large Intestine

TARGET AREAS

- Abdominals
- Hamstrings

LEGS UP THE WALL (YIN)

WHAT TO DO

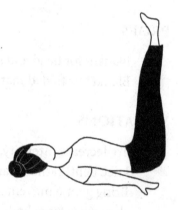

- Begin by lying down on side with bottom against wall
- Gently swing legs up against wall, legs straight over head, and wiggle until hips are square to wall and as close to wall as possible
- Allow arms to rest at sides, palms facing up
- Allow neck to be neutral (can have a blanket underneath neck and head)
- Rest here, breathing slowly and evenly as you hold pose for one to ten minutes or as long as comfortable
- To release pose, gently lower feet to chest and roll onto side, then come back to sitting

PROPS

- Blanket under neck/shoulders/head
- Bolster under hips

VARIATIONS

- To reduce stretch or strain on back of legs:
    - Bend knees slightly
    - Wiggle so hips are a few inches away from wall
    - Use chair/couch
- Leg variations include:
    - Feet together
    - Feet hip-width apart
    - Feet and legs in Butterfly position
    - Feet wide apart in Straddle

BENEFITS

- Restful inversion
- Decompresses and releases sacroiliac joint (SI)
- Stretches hamstrings and glutes

CAUTIONS

- Hip injuries
- Hamstring injury

MERIDIANS

- Kidney/UB

TARGET AREAS

- Spine
- Hamstrings

MEDITATION (SEATED POSITION)

WHAT TO DO

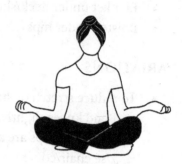

- Sit in a comfortable position, either sitting cross-legged, one or both legs outstretched on floor, or in chair. If seated in chair, try to sit slightly away from back of chair to remain upright.
- Keep eyes closed but avoid squeezing eyes shut, or keep eyes open and maintain soft or unfocused gaze on floor six to eight feet in front
- Sit up tall with spine straight, shoulders relaxed and chest open.
- Slightly tuck chin in so that head remains in line with spine
- Begin to lengthen neck and crown of head toward ceiling as if there was a golden cord attached to top of head, gently pulling head up
- To release tension in face and jaw, keep jaw slightly open and press tongue against roof of mouth
- Rest hands on knees with palms facing up
- Can lightly touch index finger to the thumb
- Relax face, jaw, and belly. Let tongue rest on roof of mouth, just behind front teeth. Allow eyes to lightly close or keep soft gaze at a point on floor about six feet ahead; let the eyes remain unfocused, eyelids heavy
- Breathe slowly, smoothly, and deeply in and out through nose. Let inhale start in belly and rise gently up into chest
- Feel breath move in and out of body, through nose, chest, lungs, and belly. Feel body as it rises and falls with each breath. Bring as much of awareness and attention to body and breath as possible with each moment
- As thoughts return to the mind, let them go, and return focus back to the body and breath

PROPS

- Cushion under sitting bones
- Blocks under knees
- Chair
- Bench for kneeling version

VARIATIONS

- Seated in chair:
  - Sit with straight back and feet flat on floor. They should form a 90-degree angle with knees. Scoot to edge of chair if necessary
  - Sit up straight, so that head and neck are in line with spine
  - Relax hands on lap (palms up or down)
- Standing:
  - Stand tall with feet shoulder-width apart
  - Shift feet so that heels turn slightly inward, and toes are pointing slightly away from each other
  - Once in position, slightly bend knees
  - Allow body to root down through feet with each exhale. Imagine energy lifting out through crown of head with each inhale
  - For added relaxation, place hands on belly to feel breath moving through body
- Kneeling:
  - Rest on floor on bent knees. Shins should be flat on floor with ankles below your bottom
  - Place cushion between bottom and heels for more support and less strain on knees (or use meditation bench)
  - Position should not be painful. If it is, try another meditation pose that is pain-free and allows for relaxation
  - Root weight back and down through hips. This prevents too much pressure on knees
- Lying down:
  - Lie on back with arms extended alongside body
  - Place feet hip-distance apart and turn out toes to side
  - If this is uncomfortable, modify pose to support lower back by placing a blanket or bolster underneath knees to slightly elevate them while lying flat, or bend knees and place feet flat on ground

BENEFITS

- Mental clarity
- Sense of calm/ease
- Parasympathetic nervous system activation (produces a sense of relaxation)
- Improved heart rate variability (HRV)
- Compassion/self-care

CAUTIONS

- Can create more stress if sympathetic nervous system is over-activated
- Eyes closed can be triggering (especially with history of trauma)
- Tingling in feet (feeling like feet have fallen asleep)

MERIDIANS

- Kidney/UB (seated)
- Liver/Gallbladder (seated)

TARGET AREAS

- Spine
- Hips
- Knees

MOUNTAIN (YANG)

WHAT TO DO

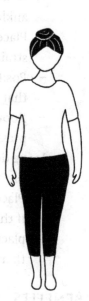

- Begin standing with feet parallel, heels slightly apart
- Focus on standing evenly on all four corners of feet (balls, toes, outer and inner edges)
- Allow thigh muscles to be active without locking knees
- Feel lift through core and up through crown of head
- Keep chin parallel to mat, creating length through neck
- Gaze forward as chest opens and shoulder blades release and draw back slightly
- Allow arms to remain naturally by sides
- Keep eyes, tongue, and facial muscles soft and relaxed
- Breathe slowly and evenly

PROPS

- Chair for Seated Mountain version

VARIATIONS

- To increase comfort, bring feet hip-width apart rather than together
- To increase intensity, place arms overhead or extend straight forward from shoulders
- Close eyes to deepen awareness and challenge balance
- To do seated in chair, actively engage leg muscles by pressing both feet evenly into floor and bringing arms overhead

BENEFITS

- Strengthens front of thighs (quadriceps)
- Strengthens core (including abdominals and muscles supporting spine)
- Strengthens shoulders (with arms overhead)
- Improves balance and focus

CAUTIONS

- Shoulder injuries
- Knee injuries (be careful not to lock knees)
- Lower back issues

MERIDIANS

- Kidney/UB
- Spleen/Stomach
- Heart/Lung/Small Intestine/Large Intestine (arms overhead version)

TARGET AREAS

- Works all major muscle groups, particularly quadriceps, core, and shoulders

QUARTER DOG (PUPPY) (YIN)

WHAT TO DO

- Begin in Tabletop and place left forearm on floor, bent perpendicular at elbow at a 90-degree angle

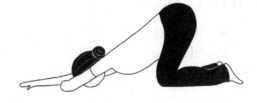

- Reach right arm above if range of motion permits, resting left elbow on floor
- Drop chest toward floor, keep hips above knees, creating arch in back
- Rest head on back of left forearm or just inside arm on floor
- Repeat on opposite side

PROPS

- Blanket/cushion under head, chest, and/or knees
- Block under hand of extended arm

VARIATIONS

- In case of shoulder sensitivity, bend extended arm at elbow
- Place block under extended arm (under forearm or hand) to raise floor
- Rest chest on bolster

BENEFITS

- Gentle inversion
- Stretches shoulders, arms (triceps), and chest
- Spinal extension (upper and middle back)

CAUTIONS

- Shoulder issues
- Knee sensitivity
- Neck pain/fragility
- Tingling in hands/fingers (could be nerve compression)

MERIDIANS

- Kidney/UB
- Spleen/Stomach
- Heart/Lung/Small Intestine/Large Intestine

TARGET AREAS

- Shoulders
- Adductors
- Spine flexion

SADDLE (YIN)

WHAT TO DO

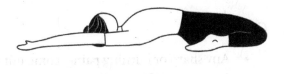

- Begin by sitting back on heels; notice sensation in knees
- If pain is present in knees, select alternative pose (Sphinx, Supported Bridge)
- If knees are comfortable, lean back on your hands and create small arch in lower back
- Remain in position or come down onto elbows or floor

PROPS

Props may be very helpful for this pose:

- Blanket under ankles or between hips and ankles for tightness
- Bolster (or two) to support torso (raising floor)
- Bolster between knees for tight ankles and hips
- Chair/couch to support back and reduce spinal extension

VARIATIONS

- To decrease intensity:
  - Try Half Saddle by straightening one leg; or bend straight leg and place foot on floor
  - Stay upright or only go as far back as elbows
  - Support back by placing bolster lengthwise under spine
  - Use one bolster or multiples, stacking two crossways under shoulders
- If there are fears/concerns about bending backward, start by leaning on chair or back of couch for support. Over time, if comfortable, attempt transition to two bolsters and eventually one
- To increase sensation, rest top of head on floor to open neck and throat
- Bring both arms overhead to open shoulders and deepen backbend

BENEFITS

- Spinal extension sacral-lumbar arch
- Stretches hips flexors and quadriceps

- Shoulder/chest opener
- Gentle inversion

CAUTIONS

- Any sharp or burning pain—come out of pose immediately
- Knees—avoid pose if knees are sensitive
- Tight ankles—use blankets or elevate hips
- Back/disc/sacrum—support spine; avoid going into extension

MERIDIANS

- Spleen/Stomach
- Kidney/UB

TARGET AREAS

- Spine extension—lumbar/sacrum
- Quadriceps, hip flexors, ankles

SAVASANA (YIN)

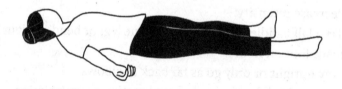

WHAT TO DO

- Begin on back and find a comfortable position with legs outstretched (place a blanket/bolster under knees to protect lower back)
- Allow feet to fall outward until knees are hip-width apart or even farther
- Bring arms to sides, palms face up or down

PROPS

- Bolster behind knees
- Blocks to support feet

- Blanket to cover body as temperature may drop when resting on the floor
- Blanket/pillow under head

VARIATIONS

- Rest in a side-lying position during later stages of pregnancy
- Legs Up the Wall for relaxing inversion

BENEFITS

- Deep rest
- Flow of energy throughout body

CAUTIONS

- Back/disc/sacrum—use knee support, use side-lying variation

MERIDIANS

- All meridians are influenced by this simple and deep relaxation

TARGET AREAS

- Spine

SEAL (YIN)

WHAT TO DO
(Similar to Sphinx pose with greater compression in spine)

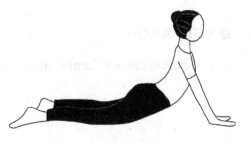

- Lie on belly, resting head on forearms
- Move elbows just ahead of shoulders, propping up trunk
- Notice sensation in lower back
- Slide hands out and lift trunk up with straight arm support (avoid locking elbows)
- Hands and arms can also turn straight out to side, more closely resembling a seal

PROPS

- Bolster or folded blanket under pubic bone can lessen the intensity in both wrists and shoulders

VARIATIONS

- To increase sensations in lower back, widen legs
- To decrease sensations along sacrum, bring legs together
- Place bolster or blanket under pubic bone or thighs to soften pressure (helpful in pregnancy)
- Relax shoulders to bring more ease to shoulders/neck

BENEFITS

- Deep compression in sacral-lumbar area of spine
- Stretch of stomach

CAUTIONS

- Back injury or back pain
- Do not stay in pose if there are any sharp pains
- Avoid full pose if pregnant
- Headaches

MERIDIANS

- Kidney/UB
- Spleen/Stomach

TARGET AREAS

- Spine extension-lumbar area

SEATED TWIST (YANG)

WHAT TO DO

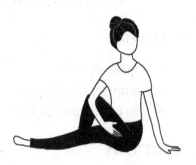

- In seated position, extend legs in front of body and sit up straight
- If hips are very tight, sit on bolster or folded blanket
- Balance weight evenly across sit bones
- Align head, neck, and spine; lengthen spine, keep neck relaxed
- Cross left leg over the outstretched right leg, just above the right knee
- Place left hand on floor behind your left hip. Bring right hand to outside of left knee
- Exhale while gently twisting to left
- Inhale again as you lengthen spine, and exhale as you twist deeper
- Gaze over left shoulder. Do not push hard against knee to force a deeper twist
- Keep collarbones broad. Sit up straight. Do not round shoulders
- Do not lean torso forward to obtain a deeper twist, only as far as possible while keeping head aligned directly over tailbone
- Exhale as you come back to center
- Recross opposite legs and repeat twist on opposite side for same length of time
- To release pose, come back to center

PROPS

- Blanket or bolster to prop hips
- Chair for seated chair version

VARIATIONS

- For tight hips, sit on blanket, pile of firm blankets, yoga bolster or block, or meditation pillow to reduce stress on hips, knees, and back, and to open groin
- Seated in chair:
  - Keep both feet flat on floor and knees facing forward
  - To twist to right, grasp back of chair with right hand and place left hand on right knee

- Release back to center
- Repeat twist on opposite side

BENEFITS

- Opens shoulders
- Improves flexibility of spine
- Decreases back stiffness

CAUTIONS

- Tight hips
- Neck strain/neck injury

MERIDIANS

- Liver/Gallbladder

TARGET AREAS

- Obliques/diaphragm muscles

SHOELACE (YIN)

WHAT TO DO

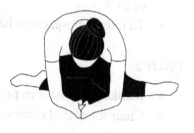

- Begin by sitting cross-legged, then draw one foot under opposite thigh and other foot across toward opposite hip
- Anchor both sitting bones to floor equally (if hips are tight, sit on blanket or bolster to tilt hips forward)
- Slide feet out next to each opposite hip as far as safely possible
- To help distribute weight evenly: fold forward, place hands on floor, or rest elbows on thighs or bolster

PROPS

- Blanket placed under hips if tight
- Folded blanket to fill space between knees or underneath bottom knee/thigh (bend or straighten leg according to preference)

- Bolster/block to rest torso or elbows in forward fold

VARIATIONS

- Half Shoelace version if knee pain or tight hips:
  - Extend one leg and bring other (bent) leg across to the outside of hip on the opposite side
  - Stack knees with option to fold forward
- For lower back pain, sit upright and bring hands to side or in front of body to put more weight on hands and arms, or reach arms behind body and lean backward
- Add lateral (side-bending) stretch from either half or full variation:
  - Place one hand on floor next to hip, sliding it away from body
  - Stretch other arm over head in same direction, with soft or stronger stretch according to preference
  - Press opposing sitting bone toward floor

BENEFITS

- Hip opener (both for top and bottom hips)
- Spinal flexion when taking forward fold
- Stomach compression

CAUTIONS

- Knee pain
- Can aggravate sciatica
- Lower back pain

MERIDIANS

- Liver/Gall bladder
- Kidney/UB

TARGET AREAS

- Glutes
- Spine flexion

SIDE-LYING BANANA (YIN)

WHAT TO DO

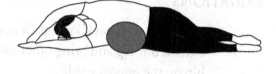

- Place bolster to your right side. Roll over it so bolster is under right armpit and right side of rib cage (bolster is horizontal rather than vertical on mat)
- Bend knees to side and come into side-lying position
- To deepen stretch, extend right arm on floor and rest head on right bicep
- Rest left arm alongside of body, or reach it overhead and bring left and right palms together
- To switch sides, come into side-lying position on right side and roll over to left, adjusting position on bolster as necessary

PROPS

- Bolster for side stretch
- Blanket between knees
- Block for bottom arm
- Block for head

VARIATIONS

- To increase sensations, straighten top leg and reach through toes with bottom knee bent, or reach top leg back on diagonal
- To decrease sensations, lower top arm to your side and rest it there; or if keeping arm overhead, rest it on a block

BENEFITS

- Deep lateral (side) stretch
- Helps decrease shallow breathing by opening tight intercostal muscles
- Reduces stiffness and tension around neck, shoulders, upper back
- Stretches abdominal muscles

CAUTIONS

- Shoulder pain/injury
- Hip pain

MERIDIANS

- Liver/Gallbladder

TARGET AREAS

- Arms/shoulders
- Upper back
- Chest

SLEEPING SWAN (PIGEON) (YIN)

WHAT TO DO

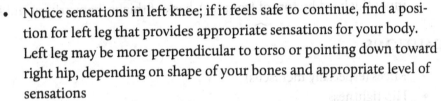

- Begin in Tabletop or Down Dog
- Draw left knee to left wrist and place left ankle down toward front of right hip
- Notice sensations in left knee; if it feels safe to continue, find a position for left leg that provides appropriate sensations for your body. Left leg may be more perpendicular to torso or pointing down toward right hip, depending on shape of your bones and appropriate level of sensations
- Tuck right toes under and slide right knee away from body, straightening back leg
- Lower hips to floor, right toes pointing away, kneecap and top of foot resting on floor
- To lift torso away from ground, press through fingertips, lengthening front of body (Upright Swan)
- Try to balance weight evenly between left and right hips; use a blanket if needed under left hip to balance weight or relieve tightness in left hip
- Slowly walk hands forward on mat
- Torso remains upright with hands on mat for support; or lower torso onto forearms or elbows; or if range of motion permits, lower chest to floor
- Repeat on opposite side

PROPS

- Blanket/bolster under one or both hips to support the hips
- Bolster lengthwise under the chest

VARIATIONS

- If flexible, draw front foot forward, bring front knee out to side, and rest chest on top of shin
- To increase sensation, add a twist by reaching arm (same side as the front leg) under torso and extend as far as range of motion permits
- Deer pose or Figure Four are alternatives that provide similar benefit to target area of hips/quads

BENEFITS

- Strengthens muscles supporting spine, abdominals (eccentrically), back of thighs (hamstrings), buttocks (gluteal and deeper muscles like piriformis), chest, arms, shoulders
- Stretches abdominals, shoulders, front of hips (hip flexors of back leg), inner thigh (adductors of front leg), back of thighs (hamstrings), ankles

CAUTIONS

- Knees (especially meniscus)
- Hip tightness

MERIDIANS

- Liver/Gallbladder
- Spleen/Stomach
- Kidney/UB

TARGET AREAS

- Glutes
- Psoas
- Hip flexors
- Spinal extension (upright position)
- Spinal flexion (forward fold position)

SNAIL (YIN)

WHAT TO DO

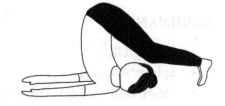

- Lie on back, hands alongside body
- Inhale, bend knees, and bring feet over head toward floor
- Try to position weight of body mostly in shoulders, rather than neck
- If feet can reach floor, round back as you bend, and lower knees alongside ears as feet fall toward floor
- If feet do not reach floor, support lower back with hands
- To come out of pose, try to keep knees bent; hold hips and slowly roll down. Okay if head lifts a little as you come down; try to land gently on back while descending

PROPS

- Blocks/bolsters to rest feet after bringing them over head
- Folded blanket beneath the shoulders to protect neck

VARIATIONS

- If feet do not reach floor, support lower back with palms of hands
- Plow version: Keep legs straight (either touching floor or keeping hands on lower back)

BENEFITS

- Elongates tissues in back
- Relaxes heart and brings more blood flow to head
- Provides stimulating chest and abdominal compression

CAUTIONS

- Neck sensitivity
- High blood pressure
- Eye issues
- Lower back issues
- Pregnancy

- Nausea/vertigo
- Sinus issues, head cold, etc.

MERIDIANS

- Kidney/UB
- Spleen/Stomach
- Heart/Lung/Small Intestine/Large Intestine

TARGET AREAS

- Stretches the entire spine
- Strengthens shoulders

SPHINX (YIN)

WHAT TO DO

- Lie down on belly with legs extended behind you, hip-width apart
- Relax the buttocks
- Bring arms up and rest elbows just in front of shoulders with forearms parallel to each other
- Press forearms down on mat and lift chest and head away from the floor to create a small backbend

PROPS

- Bolster or folded blanket under pubic bone
- Cushion or bolster under arms

VARIATIONS

- To decrease sensation, slide elbows further away to reduce compression in lower back
- To reduce compression even further, simply lie on stomach
- To deepen sensations in lower back, elevate elbows or chest on a cushion

- Place bolster under armpits and allow chin and forehead to rest on top of bolster
- To protect lower back, engage buttocks and inner thighs

BENEFITS

- Promotes tissue health along spine
- Possible therapeutic effects for chronic back/disc issues

CAUTIONS

- Acute back/disc injuries

MERIDIANS

- Kidney/UB

TARGET AREAS

- Lumbar spine extension

SQUARE (YIN)

WHAT TO DO

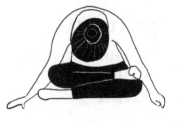

- Start seated and straighten right leg out and place left ankle under right knee
- Bend right knee and draw right foot in on top of left knee (left foot remains in same place)
- Rest forward if able, or stay upright
- Repeat on opposite side

PROPS

- Folded blanket under hips to help deepen forward fold; or use to fill in space between top knee and bottom ankle to allow top leg to feel supported
- Bolster to rest upper body/torso in forward fold

VARIATIONS

- If knees/hips are tight, bring top foot in front of bottom knee on floor (Open Square)
- To increase sensation, draw knees closer together, pushing feet further apart
- Other alternatives: Deer, Figure Four, or Shoelace/Half Shoelace

BENEFITS

- Bilateral external rotation for hips, allowing for deep hip opener
- Spinal flexion in forward fold expression

CAUTIONS

- Pressure on knees (especially with hip tightness)
- Tight ankles (for top foot)
- Can aggravate sciatica
- Lower back issues

MERIDIANS

- Liver/Gallbladder
- Kidney/UB

TARGET AREAS

- Iliotibial (IT) band
- Hips
- Spine

SQUAT (YANG)

WHAT TO DO

- Stand with feet hip-width apart
- Gently ease down into squat by bending knees and find appropriate level of sensation, making sure that knees and feet are pointing in same direction

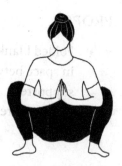

- Bring arms in front, palms together, and elbows lightly rest against knees or shins; or rest hands on floor

PROPS

- Block to sit on
- Folded blanket or bolster beneath heels

VARIATIONS

- If ankles are tight and/or heels are off floor, place folded blanket under them
- If knees are sensitive, stay upright in a modified squat, resting elbows on thighs
- For more ease, relaxation, and support, sit on a block and/or sit against wall
- To increase sensation, explore taking feet wider apart to deepen hip opener
- Deepen level of sensation by keeping feet together and knees wide apart; wrap arms around shins and clasp hands together behind back, relaxing head and neck

BENEFITS

- Opens hips
- Strengthens ankles
- Releases lower back

CAUTIONS

- Tight hips may hinder knees from deeper bend
- Knee injuries
- Tight ankles

MERIDIANS

- Liver/Gallbladder
- Kidney/UB

TARGET AREAS

- Spine

- Groin
- Ankles
- Glutes

STANDING HALF-MOON OR SEATED HALF-MOON (CRESCENT MOON) (YANG)

WHAT TO DO

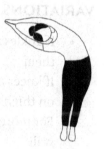

- Begin by standing in Mountain pose
- Interlace fingers, pointing index finger up over head
- Press feet into floor and reach up with fingers and crown of head
- Relax shoulders back and down to avoid neck/shoulder tension
- Exhale and press right hip out to side, arching over to left
- Keep feet grounded and evenly distribute weight in both legs
- Release by inhaling and reaching fingers up toward ceiling again
- Keeping arms up, repeat on other side
- Lower arms down after comleting both sides

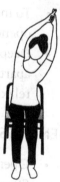

PROPS

- Chair for seated version

VARIATIONS

- Bring feet wider apart
- If shoulders are injured, sensitive, or have limited range of motion, place lower hand on hip and extend just higher arm toward opposite side

BENEFITS

- Stretches and opens side body
- Stretches shoulders
- Improves core/abdominal strength

- Strengthens ankles and knees

CAUTIONS

- Shoulder injury
- Hip injury
- Back pain

MERIDIANS

- Liver/Gallbladder
- Heart/Lung/Small Intestine/Large Intestine

TARGET AREAS

- Ankles/knees
- Shoulders
- Abdominals/obliques

TABLETOP/EXTENDED TABLETOP (YANG)

TABLETOP

WHAT TO DO

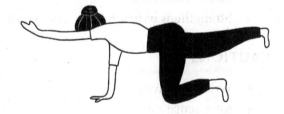

- Come to floor on hands and knees
- Bring knees hip-width apart, with feet directly behind knees
- Bring palms directly under shoulders with fingers facing forward
- Look down between palms and flatten back
- Press palms into floor to drop shoulders slightly away from ears
- Press tailbone toward back wall and crown of head toward front wall to lengthen spine

EXTENDED TABLETOP

WHAT TO DO

- From Tabletop, extend the right leg behind you at hip level
- Keep the spine neutral and engage abdominal muscles
- Extend left arm out in front of you at shoulder level and reach through your fingertips
- Keep hips level by pointing the right foot down toward the ground
- Hold for a count of 3 to 5 breaths
- Repeat on the other side

PROPS

- Place folded blanket under knees

VARIATIONS

- If wrists are sensitive, make fists to reduce pressure or come onto forearms

BENEFITS

- Stable posture to help lengthen spine
- Helpful transition for many floor poses
- Strengthens core
- Strengthens wrists, fingers, and hands

CAUTIONS

- Wrist sensitivity
- Knee sensitivity

MERIDIANS

- Kidney/UB

TARGET AREAS

- Hands/wrists
- Knees
- Spine

THREAD THE NEEDLE (YANG)

WHAT TO DO

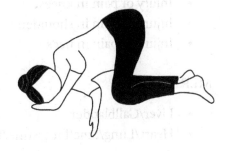

- Begin on hands and knees in Tabletop pose
- Slide right hand between left hand and left knee
- Continue to slide right arm all the way out to left so that right shoulder and side of head rest comfortably on floor
- Remain here, or inhale and reach left hand up toward the ceiling
- Explore appropriate stretch, then stay in it and reach out through fingers
- To release: Exhale palm back to floor and slowly inhale back to Table pose
- Repeat on the other side

PROPS

- Blanket under knees
- Blanket under shoulder/side of head that is resting on floor

VARIATIONS

- To increase shoulder opening, bring upper hand over back and hold onto inside of opposite thigh
- To challenge balance, raise top leg off ground along with top arm or bend top leg and reach for ankle/foot to come into a half bow position to stretch quadricep muscle of bent leg
- To decrease intensity, keep top hand on floor, elbow bent at a 90-degree angle

BENEFITS

- Stretches shoulders
- Stretches arms
- Stretches upper back and neck
- Engages and strengthens core and balance

CAUTIONS

- Injury or pain in knees
- Injury or pain in shoulders
- Injury or pain in neck

MERIDIANS

- Liver/Gallbladder
- Heart/Lung/Small Intestine/Large Intestine

TARGET AREAS

- Shoulders
- Hips
- Spine

TWIST (RECLINING) AND TWISTED ROOT (YIN)

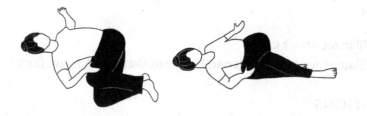

WHAT TO DO

- Begin on back with knees drawn into chest
- Open both arms out to side (like an airplane or bird wings), palms facing up or down
- Drop both knees to one side
- Support opposite shoulder with blanket if it is lifting off floor
- Gaze up at ceiling or away from knees
- Repeat on opposite side

PROPS

- Blanket/bolster beneath knees if they don't reach floor
- Blanket if shoulder is floating off floor when opposite knee is on floor

VARIATIONS

- Knees can be directed in different positions to influence stretch along spine. Bring knees higher toward chest to move twist into upper back. Lower knees toward pelvis to experience more sensation in the lumbar/sacrum area of the back
- To increase sensations along back, use opposite hand (drawn across body), traction knee away from body, and deepen twist
- Straighten arm opposite knees for shoulder opening
- Twisted Root variation: Start on back and cross one knee over other (as in Eagle) and arms out to the sides for support. While keeping upper body/shoulders rooted to floor, allow knees to fall over to floor on one side, still maintaining connection with legs wrapped together (knees crossed one on top of the other)
- Twisted-Twisted Variation: From Twisted Root position with one knee crossed over the other on the floor to one side, draw legs back up, maintaining wrapped position, and allow knees to rest on other side (same side as top leg)

BENEFITS

- Stretches tissues all along spine and releases tension
- Can reduce sciatica
- Internal massage of stomach and digestive organs

CAUTIONS

- Shoulder issues
- Tingling in hands when extended overhead
- Tight hips/hip injury
- Lower back injury

MERIDIANS

- Liver/Gallbladder
- Heart/Lung/Small Intestine/Large Intestine

TARGET AREAS

- Spine
- Shoulders
- Obliques
- Iliotibial band/Glutes

Chapter 16

PRACTICES FOR EMOTIONAL WELL-BEING

The following sequences are designed to provide suggestions of practices to use for different mental health conditions discussed in this book, and they correspond accordingly with various chapters. They are not prescriptive in any way, and any yoga teacher, therapist, or other professional who utilizes these practices should do so only with sufficient training and/or supervision from an experienced yoga professional. Before starting a new physical practice, including yoga, individuals should always get medical clearance from their physician.

SEQUENCES FOR CHAPTER 3: YIN YOGA FOR PERSONAL PRACTICE (INCLUDING SELF-INQUIRY SEQUENCES)

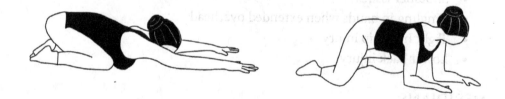

YIN POSE: WIDE-KNEE CHILD OR FROG
This pose can be done in either Wide-Knee Child or Frog. If you are newer to the practice, begin with Wide-Knee Child.

- Begin in a comfortable seated position
- Scan the body for any sensations that you notice
- Bring attention to breath and take next 1–2 minutes simply noticing

the breathing. Pay attention to where the sensations of breath are most predominant (e.g., warmth at the nostrils, abdomen rising/falling)
- Prepare for Wide-Knee Child pose, using supports to make pose safe and comfortable for the body; for example, spreading a blanket on mat so knees have some padding
- Bring knees as wide as they can go on the mat. Bring hips back toward knees as far as knees are comfortable. Hips can also remain in line with knees if there is knee discomfort. Lower torso down to mat

Initial inquiry: Notice sensations present right now in the body and begin to observe them.

- Where are they located?
- What is quality of sensations?
- Do they connect to specific emotions?
- Without judgment, really notice physical experience in present moment (for example, feeling tightness in abdomen)
- Using yin sensation scale, select current number that best represents sensations right now
- Gently try to intensify sensations just one or two numbers higher on the scale, either by either drawing knees further apart on mat, or lengthening spine
- What happens with increased sensations?
- Describe thoughts, feelings, emotions, and breath
- Try to reduce amount of sensation, just by one or two numbers, and notice how that affects you

Now, choose the amount of sensation you are comfortable with and continue to practice with what is coming up moment to moment, remaining curious.

- If you become overwhelmed or distracted, go back to the breath and use as an anchor for staying present
- Come out of pose when you have completed ten breaths
- Pause and take a moment to reflect on the following for the second inquiry:
  - What sensations did I experience in initial pose?
  - How did sensations change as I increased intensity?
  - Any thoughts/feeling/emotions that came up in the pose?
  - Did they change as accompanying sensations changed?

- What happened to sensations over time—at five breaths, at ten breaths?
- What was quality of my attention? Focused, distracted, intermittent?

SEQUENCES FOR CHAPTER 4: YIN YOGA PRACTICES FOR NERVOUS SYSTEM REGULATION

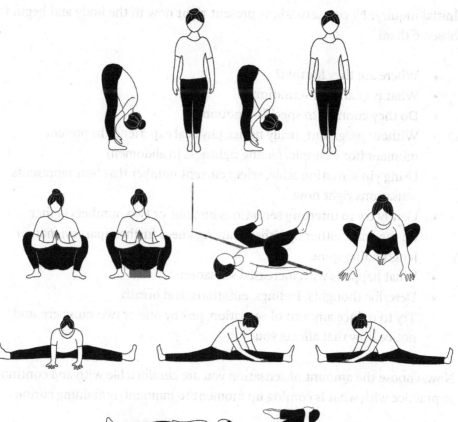

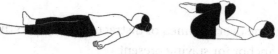

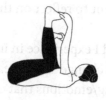

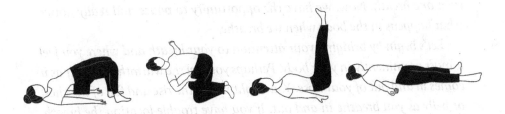

The three basic platforms that underlie a comprehensive approach to Yin yoga are meditation, breath movement and regulation (*pranayama*), and yoga postures (*asana*). Each practice I provide in this book will contain these three elements, customized to address specific emotional and behavioral issues. The following practice is for nervous system regulation.

MEDITATION: AWARENESS OF BREATH

Breath awareness can support self-regulation and reduce anxiety, depression, irritability, muscle tension, headaches, and fatigue. We often start with this simple practice of breath awareness because developing a full meditation practice can be challenging for people, especially if they have difficulty with nervous system regulation. Asking an anxious person to sit quietly and do "nothing" can be like expecting a puppy not to move when it sees another dog. This simple meditation of breath awareness can be practiced with ease and provide a sense of immediate relief and some degree of mastery. This short practice, lasting anywhere from three to ten minutes, can establish a platform of nervous system stability prior to a yin yoga practice or can help deepen a sense of safety and stability at the end of a yin yoga sequence.

AWARENESS OF BREATH SCRIPT

This simple practice allows us to reconnect to the present moment by using the anchor of the breath to help steady the mind, relax the body, and let go of mental processing. This practice can be done prior to a yoga practice or anytime throughout the day as way of taking a mindful pause.

Find a quiet place to settle in and take a few minutes to be still. Congratulate yourself for giving yourself some time to relax and reconnect to the present moment through this simple meditation practice. You can keep the eyes open or closed. If you keep your eyes open, simply lower them and allow them to soften so that you are not fixating on any one point.

Begin by simply noticing the fact that you are breathing. We breathe between 17,280 to 23,040 times a day,[1] but we often do not pay attention to even one breath. Now, we have the opportunity to pause and really notice what happens in the body when we breathe.

Let's begin by bringing your attention to your breath and where you feel it most prominently in your body. Perhaps you feel the warmth of the air as it comes in and out of your nose. You might notice the rise and fall of the chest or belly as you breathe in and out. If you have trouble locating the breath, place a hand on the stomach and the chest and just notice how the breath moves your hand.

Try to breathe naturally without trying to change the breath in any way. Simply be aware of inhaling and exhaling; breathing in and breathing out. See if you can maintain this awareness for the next several breaths in a row.

Let go of any worries, thoughts about what you are going to be doing next, or constrictions in the body. Simply watch the flow of breath, ebbing and flowing like waves in the ocean. There is no need to do anything. Just be mindful of breathing in and out. As you breathe in and out, be mindful of the chest rising on the inhalation and falling on the exhalation. Just ride the waves of the breath, moment by moment, breathing in and breathing out.

When your mind wanders away from the breath, which it may do from time to time, just simply notice where your attention went. You might note and acknowledge "thinking" or "worrying," and then gently return to the next breath. Breathing naturally and normally, observe the inhale, the exhale, and the space before the next breath.

As you come to the end of this meditation, acknowledge your act of kindness and self-love. You have taken an important step in learning how to be present in the here and now.

BREATH MOVEMENT

This form of breath movement or breath regulation is known as *pranayama* in yoga. This is a Sanskrit word: *prana* is translated as "life force," "energy," or "breath sustaining the body"; *ayama* is translated as "control" or "extend." Taken together, *pranayama* can be defined as voluntary breath control. There is a growing body of research suggesting that *pranayama* breathing can positively impact the nervous system, making the parasympathetic nervous system more dominant. Specifically, researchers and mental health clinicians have been focused on how the impact of intentional slow deep breathing, often referred to as conscious or coherent breathing, can be utilized to treat different nervous system disorders.

Slow conscious breathing is one of the foundations of yin yoga, as it allows students to begin to take control of their nervous system responses even before they do a yin pose. When we don't attempt to regulate our breathing, the nervous system can easily go into hypoarousal mode, particularly if it is already in a more chronically stressed state. I like to spend several minutes doing this slow breathing practice, which can amplify the sense of relaxation throughout the yin practice.

CONSCIOUS BREATHING SCRIPT

This simple breath practice can help you to feel more relaxed, alert, and able to focus. By regularly slowing the breath down and creating balance in your inhalation and exhalation, you will feel how the body naturally begins to let go and find ease. Practice conscious breathing from five minutes to 20 minutes. It can be practiced as a stand-alone pranayama practice or as part of a yin yoga practice.

Slowly close the eyes, or keep a soft gaze with the eyes relaxed and not fixated on any one point. Begin to focus on your breathing without the intention to change it in any way. Simply pay attention to the breath and notice the physical sensations associated with breathing, including the belly and chest rising and falling, the air moving in and out of the nose or mouth. Stay with this for several rounds of breath.

After these initial rounds of natural breathing, bring awareness to the qualities of your breath. If possible, continue to gently breathe in and out through the nose. As you breathe in and out through the nose, start to count the length of the inhalation. Notice how may beats or counts it takes to fully inhale. Do not change the breath, simply notice the length of the in-breath.

Notice the exhalation next. Notice how many beats or counts it takes to fully exhale. You may notice that your inhale or exhale is longer. This is not a problem. You are simply noticing the natural ratio of inhalation to exhalation.

Now, notice the quality of the inhalation. Is it full and deep, expanding both your belly and chest, or more shallow and limited to only the chest? Now, notice the quality of the exhalation. Does the chest and belly slowly fall and relax on the exhalation, or does the breath exit the chest only? Notice if there are pauses between the inhalation and exhalation, both at the top of the inhalation and the bottom of the exhalation.

Now, see if you can begin to find a smooth rhythmic quality to the breath. Concentrate on expanding the belly and chest on the in-breath and allowing the chest and belly to empty and relax on the out-breath.

After a few minutes, begin to lengthen both the inhalation and exhalation. The lengthening should be gradual, one or two beats at most. See how this feels. If it feels comfortable, continue to stay with this extended breathing.

See if you can regulate the breath so that the inhalation and exhalation are the same length now. It is important not to force the breathing in any way. Forcing the breath can actually tighten the muscles that help us to breathe (diaphragm, face, and neck) and can create stress in the nervous system. Back off by one or more beats if the breathing starts to feel labored or difficult in any way. Once you have found a comfortable rhythm, stay with this practice of equal inhalation and exhalation or 1:1 ratio breath for up to five minutes. Slowly open your eyes and notice how you feel. Congratulate yourself for giving yourself the time to soothe the nervous system and increase your sense of well-being.

POSTURE FLOW FOR NERVOUS SYSTEM REBALANCE
YIN SEQUENCE

- Dangle (Standing forward fold)—2 min.
- Mountain—2 min.
- Repeat first two poses
- Squat (variations using blocks; wall) or Seated Butterfly—2 min.
- Dragonfly—lateral (both sides) and forward fold—15 min. total
- Rest on back—2 min.
- Legs into chest—3 min.
- Stirrup (variations: Frog inversion; Butterfly inversion)—5 min.
- Supported Bridge—5 min.
- Reclining Twist (both sides)—10 min. total
- Legs Up the Wall—5 min.
- Relaxation—5 to 15 min.

SEQUENCES FOR CHAPTER 5: YIN YOGA AND POSITIVE EMOTIONS (WITH YIN/YANG FLOW)

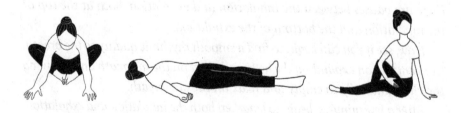

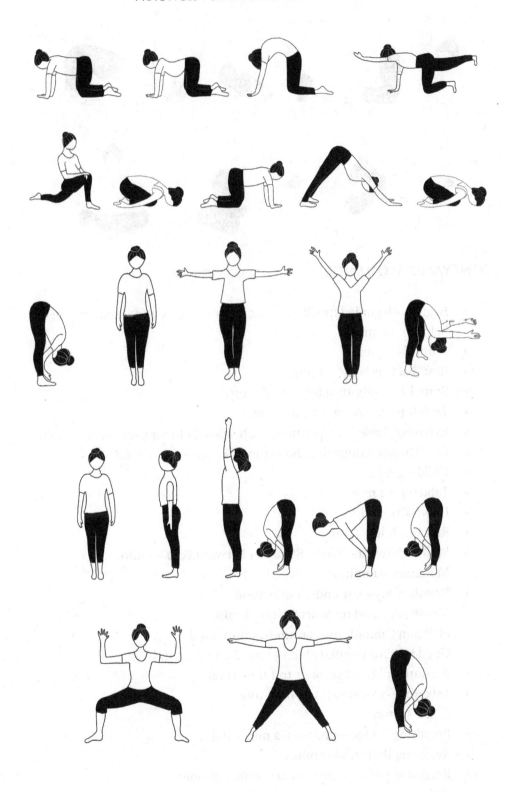

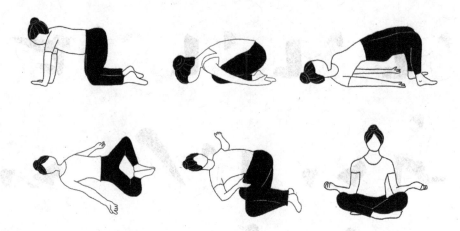

YIN/YANG SEQUENCE

- Begin with guided meditation for inner resource and intention (see below)—10 min.
- Butterfly—5 min.
- Rest (back or belly)—2 min.
- Seated Twist (both sides)—4 min. total
- Tabletop—Cat/Cow—2 min. flow
- Extended Table—5 repetitions each side—hold for 5 sec.; rest for 30 sec.
- Easy Dragon Lunge (hands on top of knee)—4 min. total
- Child—2 min.
- Tabletop—1 min.
- Down Dog—1 min.
- Rest in Child—1 min.
- Walk feet toward hands, Standing Forward Fold—1 min.
- Mountain—1 min.
- Breath of Joy—5 rounds, 2 min. total
- Mountain (hand on heart/belly)—1 min.
- Half Sun Salutations—5 rounds, 5 min. total
- Goddess/Five-Pointed Star—5 rounds, 2 min. total
- Forward Fold—30 seconds to 1 min. total
- Tabletop—30 seconds to 1 min. total
- Child—1 min.
- Breathing Bridge—5 rounds, 2 min. total
- Reclining Butterfly—3 min.
- Reclining Twist—6 min. total (3 min. per side)
- Guided meditation—5 to 15 min. lovingkindness (see below)

SCRIPT FOR GUIDED MEDITATION FOR INNER RESOURCE AND INTENTION

Allow yourself to come into a comfortable position, either seated or lying down. Gently scan your body to see if there are any modifications or supports you need to make yourself more at ease and find even 5 or 10 percent more comfort in your body. You may want to support your back if you are resting on the earth by placing a blanket or bolster underneath your knees and place an eye pillow over your eyes. If you are sitting in a chair, you may want to place a support under your feet if they don't touch the floor, or a small cushion between your back and the chair to maintain an erect yet comfortable position.

Take a few moments to sense the room around you. Eyes can be open or closed as you open your senses. Feel the temperature of the air on your skin. Notice the support underneath you; the lighting in the room beneath your closed lids if your eyes are closed, or the colors of the room if your eyes are open.

Now begin to become aware of your intention for this practice today. (Pause here.) Consider what matters most to you right now. Focus on what would support you the most in this practice today. As you land on this intention, imagine for a moment that it has already come true and use the present tense. For example, if your intention is to feel less stress in your body, you might say, "I have ease in my body." If your intention is to feel less depressed, you might say, "The natural joy of being alive is here." Imagine how this intention can support your entire practice and even after your practice is complete. (Pause here.)

Come back to your senses once again, opening them up to what is happening in this present moment: eyes, ears, sense of touch, smell, and taste. Notice how this brings you immediately back to the present moment. This can help you any time you get distracted, overwhelmed, or tired. (Pause here.)

Let's spend some time next to develop your inner resource. An inner resource is a feeling of safety, well-being, stability, or simply feeling okay in the body. An inner resource can be cultivated through an image of beautiful scenery like the ocean, a special room in your house, a person you love who makes you feel safe and calm, or a place in your body that feels calm and relaxing, such as your belly. (Pause here.)

Once you land on your inner resource today, notice the sensations in the body that accompany this image. (Pause here.) Notice where you feel the sensations most predominantly and how they may shift as images come and go. (Pause here.) This inner resource can be a helpful anchor for your practice today and even after your practice is complete. You can come back to it if you feel anxious, overwhelmed, or just need a pause to check in with yourself.

Now for the final few moments, scan your body once more and notice how you are feeling. (Pause here.) Come back to your senses once again, opening them up to what is happening in this present moment: eyes, ears, sense of touch, smell, and taste. If your eyes are closed, you may want to slide them open and closed a few times, to allow yourself to begin to transition into full awakeness and presence.

SEQUENCES FOR CHAPTER 6: YIN YOGA AND THE BREATH PRACTICES

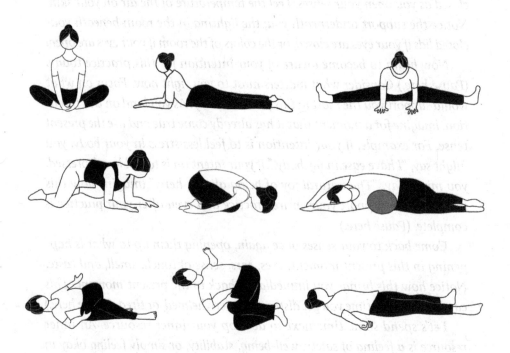

BODY SCAN MEDITATION SCRIPT

During this body scan practice, we will pay attention to the different sensations in the body as we move from one area to the other. Sensations might include temperature, pressure, tingling, tightness, numbness, or no sensation at all. There is no need to move the body part, but rather to pay attention and receive the sensations just as they are.

You can do this practice sitting up or lying down; choose a position that is most comfortable for you. Take a few moments to do a mindful check-in.

Notice any sensations in the body, thoughts that might be coming and going, and emotions that are present. Allow whatever is here to just be here, without judging, analyzing, or trying to make anything go away.

When you are ready, gently shift your focus to the breath. We will now establish a pattern of breathing that will support a calming and relaxing effect for your entire body.

Let's take two deep, relaxing breaths together. If you are able, breathe in through your nose and breathe out with a sigh. Let's do that again, breathing in and out slowly.

Now allow your eyes to soften or, if it feels more comfortable, close them. Relax the muscles around your eyes, eyebrows, and jaw. Soften your neck and shoulders, arms, and hands. Soften the muscles of your back if you can, letting go of tension starting from the top of your spine and going all the way down your back. Relax the muscles of your chest, belly, legs, and feet.

Begin to focus your attention on your breath. Breathing in and out slowly, feel the breath move in and out of your nose and throat. Taking your time, count slowly to yourself for the next few minutes.

As you breathe in, count one, two and as you breathe out, count one, two. Continue for two breaths silently to yourself. Now, count slowly to yourself as you breathe in, one, two, three, and as you breathe out, one, two, three. Practice this for three more breaths. Now, count slowly to yourself as you breathe in, one, two, three, four, and as you breathe out, one, two, three, four. Continue this for five rounds of breath, gently breathing in and softly breathing out. Now, allow your breath to find its natural rhythm, letting go of counting. Imagine your body is being breathed.

Now feel into your body lying here, relaxed and at ease. Notice where the body is being supported, feeling your back, hips, legs, and feet resting on the earth. Notice your hands, arms, and back of your head.

Starting with your feet, can you place all your attention on them? Feel into both feet, the soles of the feet, the area where your feet are touching the floor or your socks or shoes. Notice if there is tingling, coolness or warmth, or no sensation at all. Now move your attention up into your ankles and lower legs, noticing any sensations here. Do the sensations differ between the front of the legs and back of the legs? If you notice your mind has wandered at any point during this body scan, just gently return to the breath, and then go back to the body part we were just attending to. In this case, return to the lower legs.

Now, letting go of the lower legs, move the attention into your knees and upper legs where your legs join your torso, noticing what is here to be felt.

Perhaps noticing the contact beneath your legs; pressure, temperature, or numbness. Numbness also counts as a sensation. Now put all your attention into the lower trunk and the belly, up to the belly button, perhaps feeling the breath in the lower belly as you breathe in and out.

Now move your attention from the belly to the back of the body. The tailbone, the lower, middle, and upper back, feeling any and all sensations here. Allow any tightness to soften and relax if it is possible. If the sensations here or in any part of the body are intense or uncomfortable, you have two choices. One is to mindfully shift positions to find more ease in the body. The other is to stay with the sensations and allow them to be as they are, observing them and noticing the quality of the sensations—dull, throbbing, aching—and breathing in and out with the sensations, just as they are.

From here, move your attention around to the front of the body, the upper trunk, feeling the sensations of the breath as you fill the lungs when you breathe in and empty the lungs when you breathe out. Now put your full attention into your hands, feeling your hands. feeling each finger. Feel the position of your hands as they rest against the floor, the temperature and sensations.

Place your full attention on the wrists and forearms now. Notice your elbows and upper arms, observing any sensations here. If your mind wanders off, just bring it back to the breath and then start again with the upper arms. Now put your full attention into your shoulders, front and back, noticing any and all sensations here, another area that sometimes holds a lot of tension. Move into the back of your neck, your throat. Move your attention into the jaw and mouth, noticing any sensations here. Place your attention on your entire face, including your nose, cheeks, eyes, and forehead.

Now, bring your attention to include the entire body, from your head to your toes, noticing any and all sensations. Breathe in and imagine the breath moving from the crown of the head all the way down to the soles of the feet. Breathe out and imagine the breath moving up and out the crown of the head, being present with the sensations of the entire body, allowing the sensations to be just as they are. Allowing yourself to be just as you are. Begin to move the body gently, starting to transition from relaxed to awake and present. Perhaps, start by wiggling fingers and toes. Stretch the body in any way that feels supportive and nurturing. When you are ready, we will move into our first yin shape of this sequence.

This sequence is adapted from the Breath-Body-Mind™ training program created by Dr. Richard P. Brown and Dr. Patricia L. Gerbarg (see www.Breath-Body-Mind.com).[2,3]

YIN SEQUENCE WITH EMPHASIS ON BREATH PRACTICES

Begin at one minute per pose and increase up to five minutes per pose.

- Butterfly (mindfulness of the breath)
- Sphinx (basic coherent breathing using 4-4 count)
- Dragonfly (coherent breathing plus breath hold using 4-4-6-4 pattern)
- Frog (using *Kapalabhati*—gentle version)
- Child pose (mindfulness of the breath)
- Side-lying Banana-asana with bolster—both sides (coherent breathing plus breath hold 4-4-6-4 pattern)
- Twisted Root or Reclining Twist—both sides (mindfulness of breath)
- *Savasana*—5 to 15 min.

SEQUENCES FOR CHAPTER 8: YIN SEQUENCE FOR THE FOUR IMMEASURABLES

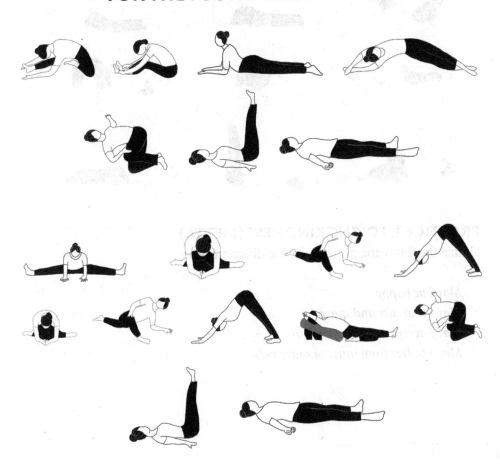

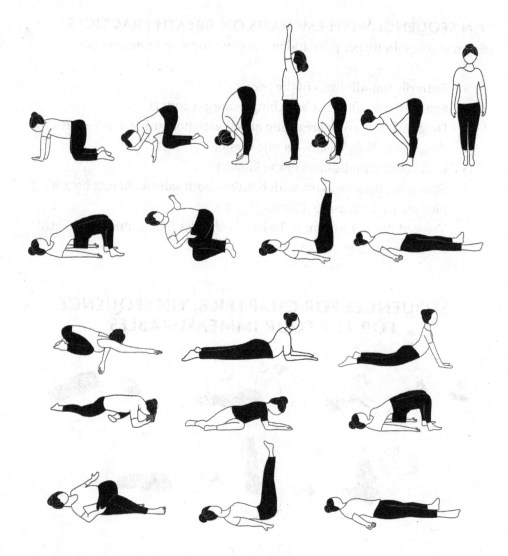

PRACTICE 1: LOVINGKINDNESS (METTA)

Utilize the following phrases during different poses:

May I be happy.
May I find ease and space.
May I accept myself just as I am.
May I be free from inner or outer pain.

SEQUENCE

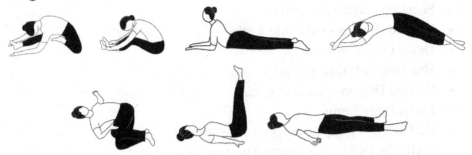

- Half Butterfly—10 min. total (5 min. per side)
- Caterpillar—5 min.
- Sphinx—5 min.
- Banana-asana—10 min. total (5 min. per side)
- Reclining Twist—10 min. total (5 min. per side)
- Meditation with Legs Up the Wall or *Savasana*—5 to 15 min. (use extended Lovingkindness meditation offered to self and others)

PRACTICE 2: COMPASSION (KARUNA)

Utilize the following phrases during different poses, particularly when challenges emerge in a pose:

I can be with this sensation for now.
I am willing to meet myself here.
I can stay here for five more breaths.
I can say yes to this even though this is difficult.

SEQUENCE

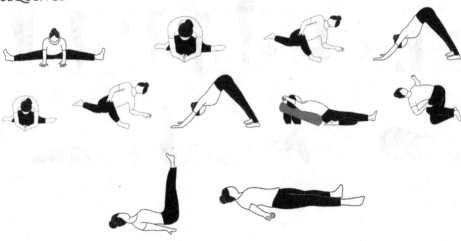

- Dragonfly—5 min.
- Shoelace—right side, 5 min.
- Winged Dragon—right side, 5 min.
- Down Dog—1 min.
- Shoelace—left side, 5 min
- Winged Dragon—left side, 5 min.
- Down Dog—1 min.
- Half Saddle—6 min. total (3 min. per side)
- Reclining Twist—10 min. total (5 min. per side)
- Meditation—5 to 15 min. in Legs Up the Wall or *Savasana* (extended Compassion meditation including both compassion for self and compassion for others)

PRACTICE 3: EMPATHETIC JOY (MUDITA) (INCLUDES YIN/YANG FLOW)

Utilize the following phrases during different poses:

I am grateful for my legs that allow me to feel the ground beneath me.
My heart is open and full.
May I feel the natural joy of being alive through this breath and these sensations.

SEQUENCE

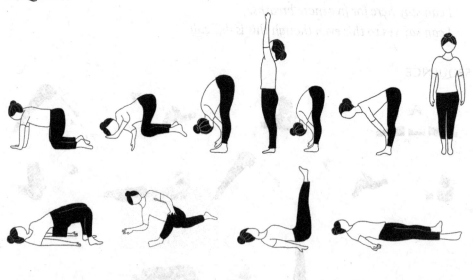

- Tabletop—1 min.
- Thread the Needle—4 min. total (2 min. per side)
- Forward Fold—1 min.
- Half Sun Salutations—5 rounds, 2 min.
- Mountain—1 min.
- Supported Bridge—5 min.
- Reclining Twist—10 min. total (5 min. per side)
- Meditation—5 to 15 min. in Legs Up the Wall or *Savasana* (extended Empathetic Joy meditation with reflection on a moment of joy experienced for others)

PRACTICE 4: EQUANIMITY (UPEKHA)

Utilize the following phrases during different poses:

I can be with this experience just as it is.
May I learn to see the changing nature of all things with equanimity and balance.
May I bring compassion and equanimity to those in need.

SEQUENCE

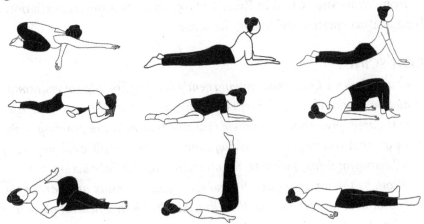

- Child with Twist—10 min. total (5 min. per side)
- Sphinx—5 min.
- Seal—2 min.
- Sleeping Swan or Deer—10 min. total (5 min. per side)
- Supported Bridge—5 min.
- Twisted Root—10 min. total (5 min. per side)
- Meditation—5 to 15 min. with Legs Up the Wall or *Savasana* (extended meditation with focus on equanimity and balance)

SEQUENCES FOR CHAPTER 9: YIN YOGA AND DBT PRACTICES (WITH SKILL-BUILDING SCRIPTS)

For additional resources on simple DBT practices, please see Marsha Linehan's workbook, *DBT Skills Training Handouts and Worksheets*[4] and Sheri Van Dijk's book, *DBT Made Simple.*[5]

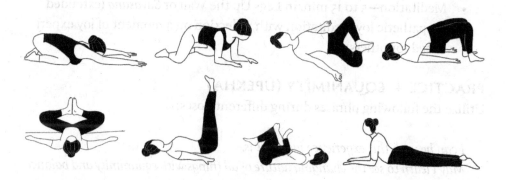

The following three scripts, **REST**, **Radical acceptance,** and **Using the senses**, can be used independently or together as a sequence. To use as a sequence, move from Wide-Knee Child in REST to Frog (or an appropriate variation) for both Radical acceptance and Using the senses.

REST SCRIPT

Take a Wide-Knee Child pose, moving gently into the first edge of your range of motion. Notice if you feel a reflex to come out of the pose or to go deeper than the appropriate edge. To provide yourself time before responding to the messages that you might be receiving from your head, utilize the following REST acronym: Relax, Evaluate, Set an intention, and Take action.

*Begin by taking a few breaths and see if you can **relax** any part of the body that does not need to hold tension, starting with a neutral place like your hands or toes.*

***Evaluate** the sensations in the body. Notice if there are still places that you are holding on to tension and see if you can relax further by envisioning that you can breathe and release any excess discomfort in this area of the body. As you stay in the pose, notice if there are any painful sensations that require skillful attention.*

*If so, **set an intention** to support yourself with more ease in the pose. Before actually moving out of the pose, consider what supports might help, whether it be a blanket, bolster, or shifting of position (for example, moving* into a variation such as Tadpole (see description of Frog pose variations in Chapter 15 or or Wide-Knee Child)).

Once you have created an intention, **take action** and mindfully move the body in a way that is supportive and allows you to stay connected to the pose.

RADICAL ACCEPTANCE SCRIPT (FOR USE FOLLOWING REST SCRIPT OR ON ITS OWN)

Start in Frog (remain in Frog if using this script as part of a sequence) or an appropriate variation of Frog for your body. Take a few moments now to acknowledge your present situation, including the sequence of poses and movements that you have used to get into this pose, any adjustments or variations you selected, and how long you have been in this shape.

Notice if any critical or judgmental thoughts are present. Observe any inner dialogue that wants this moment to be different. If so, use one or more of these Radical acceptance phrases:

The present moment is exactly what it supposed to be, even if I am uncomfortable.
The present moment is the only moment I can control.
This moment is the result of many moments leading up to right now.
I can be with this even though I am uncomfortable.
These sensations help me to feel my body and all of its wisdom.
I can move out of the pose if I choose to.

Continue to practice accepting yourself in this moment, including both the sensations in the body and any inner dialogue happening in the mind. Utilize mindfulness of the breath and continue to relax the body as much as possible.

If the mind continues to struggle with the present-moment sensations, imagine you are in a pose that provides you with ease and relaxation and how this might help you to accept reality just as it is. Acknowledge your courage and strength to stay with discomfort.

SCRIPT FOR USING THE SENSES

Take your final expression of Frog pose. Propping as appropriate so you can stay in the pose without feeling sensations that go above a 5 on your Yin scale. Connect to the present-moment sensations in your body, any emotions that are present; any and all sensations are welcome.

Begin by opening the eyes. Take a look around the room. What do you see? Can you notice the different colors and shapes in the room? How is the light hitting certain objects?

Then focus on sounds in the room, noticing any sounds in this moment. Can you hear sounds in the distance? Is your body making any sounds that you can tune in to? Do you the notice the space between sounds?

Now observe the different physical sensations of touch. Can you feel where your body is in contact with the mat, the blanket, the floor? Notice the surface textures.

Now allow the sense doorway of smell to become part of your awareness. Are there any smells that you notice? If there is nothing that arises, perhaps recall a particular pleasant scent like a flower, a candle, warm cookies.

Now, move to the sensations related to taste. Notice any particular tastes in your mouth at the present moment. If there is nothing arising, perhaps recall something that you enjoy eating and imagine how it would feel to be tasting it. Is it sweet, sour, bitter, spicy?

Now come back into the direct sensations of the body in this pose. Starting with the left side of the body, observe tingling, pulling, or any tension. Move to the right side of the body. Where do you experience sensations there? Now scan the whole body and see if you can stay with the sensations as they come and go, just like clouds in the sky.

MINDFULNESS SKILLS

WISE MIND SCRIPT

Come into Reclining Butterfly or Supported Bridge using appropriate props to help you find ease. Turn your attention toward your breath and begin to notice the rise and fall of the abdomen as you inhale and exhale.

If it is helpful, place a hand on your abdomen right below the sternum and right above the belly button. See if you can focus on breathing fully and completely into this area. Imagine this area as your wise mind, a source of stability, calm, and strength. As you breathe in and out, let your attention stay with the very center of the wise mind by breathing slowly and fully on the inhale and gently releasing slowly and fully on the exhale.

If you notice any distracting thoughts, just allow them to come and go just like the inhale and exhale of your breath and focus back on the center of the wise mind on the next breath. Concentrate on the experience of the hand resting on your stomach supporting you to stay connected with your wise mind.

Continue to pay attention to the center of the wise mind and begin to consider any difficult experiences, thoughts, problems, or physical challenges that you may be experiencing in your life. Notice how it affects you to consider these experiences, both in terms of your body's response and also in terms of your emotions.

Turn back toward the wise mind and imagine asking the center of your wise mind, "What is the most important thing I can do about this experience or situation?" Imagine your wise mind has guidance that is intuitive, coming from the gut, that can support you in the most encouraging way.

If negative thoughts or doubts arise, just acknowledge them, and return to the center of the wise mind and the feedback you are receiving. Take a few more moments to consider if the wise mind has anything else to offer.

Then return your attention to the breath for a few more rounds of full body breathing and slowly release out of the pose, taking a few moments in a rebound.

"WHAT" SKILLS SCRIPT
Take a yin pose at the wall, either Butterfly on the Wall, Legs Up the Wall, or Figure Four.

Observe: *Notice the sensations in your body as you take the shape. Then, using the sense doorway, notice different sensations coming in through your vision, hearing, smell, and taste sensory organs. Allow this open awareness to include what is occurring outside of yourself in this moment. Expand your awareness to include thoughts, feelings, and emotions. Allow this open awareness to include what is occurring inside of you from moment to moment.*

Describe: *Now, notice when a feeling or thought arises, and instead of just noticing the rise and fall, see if you can label it: "thinking" or "a feeling is here" or "judgment is present." Try not to judge or interpret the experience, just describe what you are observing in this moment.*

Participate: *For the final moments of this pose, can you completely let yourself be with all the experiences that are coming? Imagine you are simply riding the waves of the ocean, going with the flow from moment to moment. If you need to make any adjustments to ease the body, move with the guidance of the wise mind, skillfully attending to your body to ensure you are safe. Stay for a few more breaths and then lower the legs down and allow a rebound pose.*

"HOW" SKILLS SCRIPT
Select a pose at the wall (either Butterfly on the Wall, Legs Up the Wall, or Figure Four) or go to the second side if you picked a one-sided pose like

Figure Four for the previous meditation. Take a few moments to find a place of relative ease. Notice the sensations as they arise and where you experience them most predominantly.

Nonjudgmentally: *Try not to judge the sensations or experiences as good or bad. See if you can accept them as they are. Use the yin scale of sensation to help you identify the intensity of the pose and acknowledge how the intensity feels at this moment. It's fine to acknowledge any emotional reactions but try not to judge them. You might say something like "It's just hard right now."*

One-mindfully: *Now place your awareness on the strongest sensation present. See if you can just stay with this single point of attention, letting go of distractions. Or if distractions arise, redirect gently to the strongest sensation. Try to simply be with the one thing at a time. At this moment, it is the strongest sensation that is present in this pose.*

Effectively: *Now, notice if any skillful action would be helpful as you remain in this posture. You might remind yourself of why you are doing this pose, what drew you to yin yoga, and what has been helpful in the past. What is most helpful right now?*

Now open your attention to once more include the breath, physical sensations, thoughts, emotions, and allow of them to be present for the next few moments, moving from single-point concentration to open awareness. Over the next few breaths, begin to slowly transition out of the pose and release into a rebound pose.

EMOTION REGULATION

ABC PLEASE SCRIPT

*Come into Sphinx pose and find an edge that feels one or two numbers below your customary level of intensity. For example, if you typically go toward a 4 or 5 on the yin intensity scale, explore backing off and coming back to a 2 or 3 level. **Accumulate** positive emotions by recalling how you are taking care of your body and bringing health and vitality into your whole nervous system. Now, explore moving toward more intensity, by just one to two levels. **Build mastery** by noticing how you have control over what your body does and how you choose to move it or stay. Imagine going into a more challenging pose like Seal or increasing the intensity of this current pose. How would you **Cope** ahead of time with the sensations and emotions that would accompany that change? Rehearse a plan that might be helpful to skillfully meet the moment;*

perhaps remembering that as the sensations increase, you can remain steady by focusing on the breath or that these sensations will only last for a brief amount of time. Remember that you can also come out of the pose as well or decrease the intensity at any time.

As you stay in the pose, connect with the idea of PLEASE (treating physical illness, balance eating, avoid mood-altering substances, balance sleep, and get exercise), which refers to a holistic way of taking care of your mind by taking care of your body. Imagine now how you would like to care for yourself in the most compassionate and healthy way. Begin by visualizing how you respond to your physical discomfort, pain, or illness. Consider your optimal eating to maintain your energy. If you use mood-altering substances, can you imagine a plan to reduce or eliminate them from your lifestyle? What would it be like to get an "optimal" night's sleep? How would that help you to feel more energetic? Alert? Alive? Finally, can you maintain an exercise routine that would be both enjoyable and healthy?

OPPOSITE ACTION TO CHANGE EMOTIONS

Choose a challenging pose that you have some resistance toward but can still safely stay in for at least two to five minutes. Notice as you come into the pose if there are any emotions present. Notice how that emotion may create a desire to act. For example, if fear is present, the action urge may be to avoid the experience by zoning out and focusing on something else or a strong desire to move out of the pose.

Consider the following process to stay with the experience in a new way:

Step 1: *First, identify the emotion that is present. Is it fear, irritation, sadness, blame?*

Step 2: *If there are one or more emotions present, you might ask yourself to "check the facts" and see if the emotion is justified. For example, if there is fear present that you are going to injure yourself in the pose, ask yourself if this a valid concern.*

Step 3: *Describe to yourself what your urge to action is. Perhaps in this moment, there is a strong action urge to come out of the pose to reduce the intensity, or to stop doing the practice altogether.*

Step 4: *Ask yourself if it is the most effective action for this situation or if there are other options for staying in the pose safely.*

Step 5: *Identify an opposite action to your action urge. For example, staying* *in the pose for at least five more breaths might be effective to observe the experience over time and see if there is some easing to the emotions.*

Step 6: *Stay with the pose for five breaths and evaluate the emotions and physical sensations present.*

Step 7: *Continue this process for the duration of the yin pose.*

INTERPERSONAL EFFECTIVENESS

Come into a comfortable position where you can practice a guided meditation for the next several minutes. Connect to the breath and begin to notice the inhale, the exhale, and the pause at the bottom of the breath. Maintain an alert, yet relaxed posture by relaxing your shoulders, arms, and hands, making space to breathe easily in and out of the body.

Now bring to mind a difficult interaction you had recently. Try not to focus on an interaction that caused extreme distress, but instead choose one that was mildly upsetting. Notice how you feel as you consider this interaction. Can you recall what was the hardest or most upsetting part of this interaction for you? Focus on any sensations you are experiencing in your body as you stay with this experience.

When you are ready, let's try some skills to work with these difficult feelings, using DEAR MAN, which stands for Describe, Express, Assert, Reinforce, Mindful, Appear, Negotiate.

Describe: *Imagine that the person is in front of you right now. Can you describe what happened to the person, how the situation unfolded?*

Express: *Using an "I" statement, share with this person how you feel about the situation as clearly as you can.*

Assert: *Envision asking this person for something you want or being able to set boundaries clearly so that you are not hurt again.*

Reinforce: *Reinforce the benefits of getting your needs met and how it will help you in the future, so that the person understands the importance and value of those actions to you.*

Mindful: *Stay connected to your present experience and don't go into past stories or future worries.*

Appear: *Appear confident in your interactions with that person by using speech that is direct, concrete, and easy to understand.*

Negotiate: Can you come up with a win-win situation for both of you? Perhaps ask the other person what they think would be most helpful.

Now imagine a situation where you might have hurt someone else with something you said or wrote, or with an attitude that conveyed a negative emotion. Once more, observe how you feel while you consider this difficult interaction. Can you sense any emotions present? Can you locate them in your body right now?

Now, imagine if you were to go back and have another opportunity to have this interaction, but this time using the skills of GIVE, which stands for Gentle, Interested, Validate, and Easy Manner. Imagine sharing your feelings in the gentlest way possible, expressing your feelings without verbal jabs or negative body language.

Visualize how you could let the person know that you are interested by actively listening to what they have to say. Can you validate their concerns by reflecting back what is most important for them? Image how you can use an easy manner when interacting with this person, including leaving your negative attitude or angry affect behind.

Notice how you feel after applying the skills of GIVE. Are there any sensations in the body that have changed or shifted from the original situation you reflected on? Observe without judgment if there are still areas of constriction or tension in your body.

Imagine using the skills of GIVE toward yourself now, using the most kind and gentle curiosity toward your experience.

When you are ready, take a few rounds of mindful breathing, paying attention once more to the inhale and exhale. Begin to make some mindful movements coming back to the present moment.

Please see the following references for in-depth discussion, additional practices, and variations that can be utilized both in yin yoga and off the mat:

The Dialectical Behavior Therapy Skills Workbook (2nd ed.), J. McKay, J.C. Wood, and M. Brantley (2019) Oakland, CA: New Harbinger.

DBT Skills Training Handouts and Worksheets (2nd ed.), M. Linehan (2014) New York: Guilford Press.

DBT Made Simple, S. Van Dijk (2012) Oakland, CA: New Harbinger.

SEQUENCES FOR CHAPTER 10: YIN YOGA FOR DEPRESSION

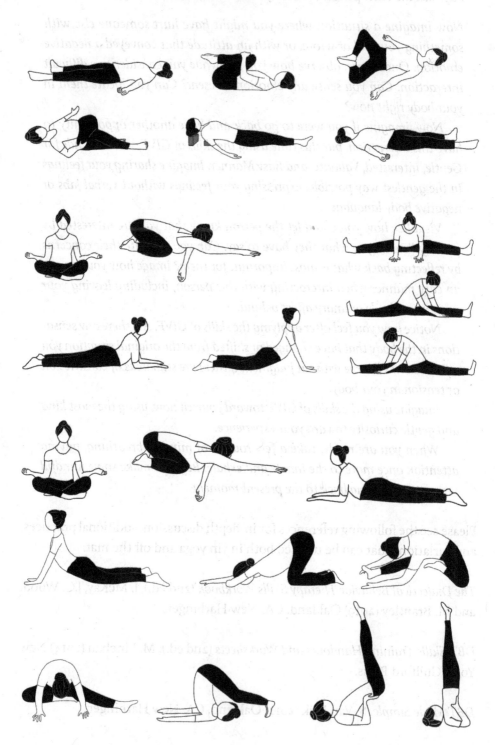

BEGINNER SEQUENCE

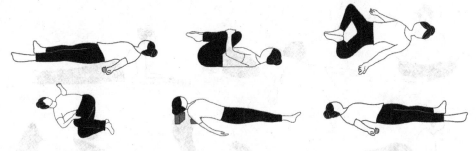

- Meditation (reclining with mindfulness of breath)—5 min.
- 3-part breath—*dirgha pranayama*
- Knees into chest—2 min.
- Reclining Butterfly—5 min.
- Reclining Twist—10 min. total (5 min. per side)
- Fish (supported with blocks)—5 min.
- *Savasana* (with guided body scan/yoga *nidra*)—5 to 15 min.

INTERMEDIATE SEQUENCE

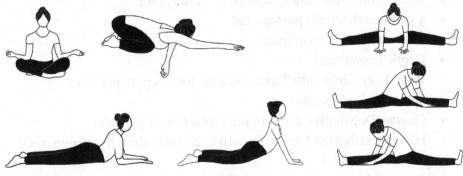

- Meditation (mindfulness of breath)—5 to 15 min.
- 3-part breath (*dirgha pranayama*)
- Alternate nostril breathing
- Wide-Knee Child with Twist—10 min. total (5 min. per side)
- Sphinx or Seal—5 min.
- Dragonfly (with option for lateral side stretch)—5 min., or 10 min. total if lateral version with 5 min. for each side

ADVANCED SEQUENCE

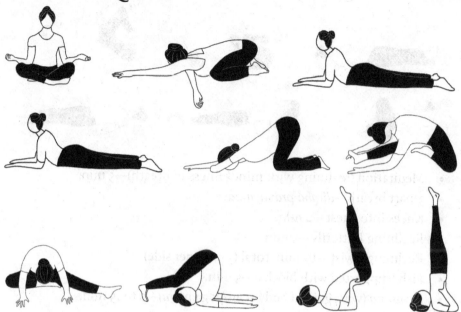

- Meditation (mindfulness of breath)—5 to 15 min.
- 3-part breath (*dirgha pranayama*)
- Alternate nostril breathing
- Gentle *kapalabhati*
- Wide-Knee Child with Twist—10 min. total (5 min. per side)
- Sphinx or Seal—5 min.
- Quarter Dog (both sides)—10 min. total (5 min. per side)
- Half Butterfly/Half Dragonfly with lateral side stretch—10 min. total (5 min. per side)
- Snail or Half Shoulder Stand/Full Shoulder Stand—5 min.

SEQUENCES FOR CHAPTER 11:
YIN YOGA FOR ANXIETY

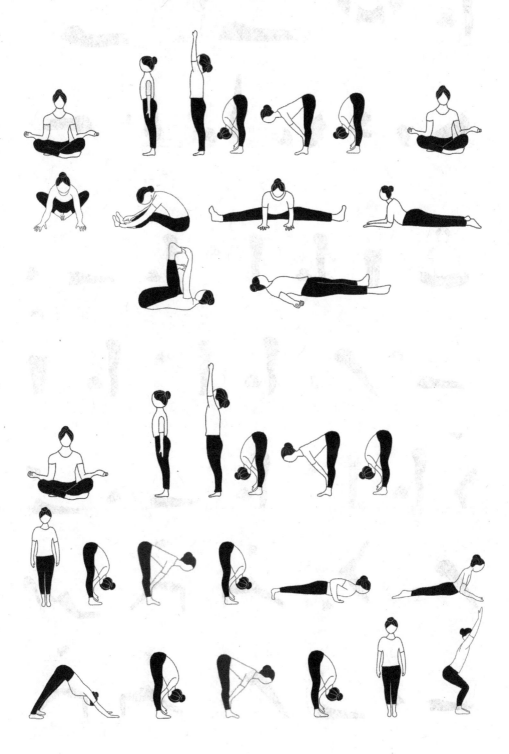

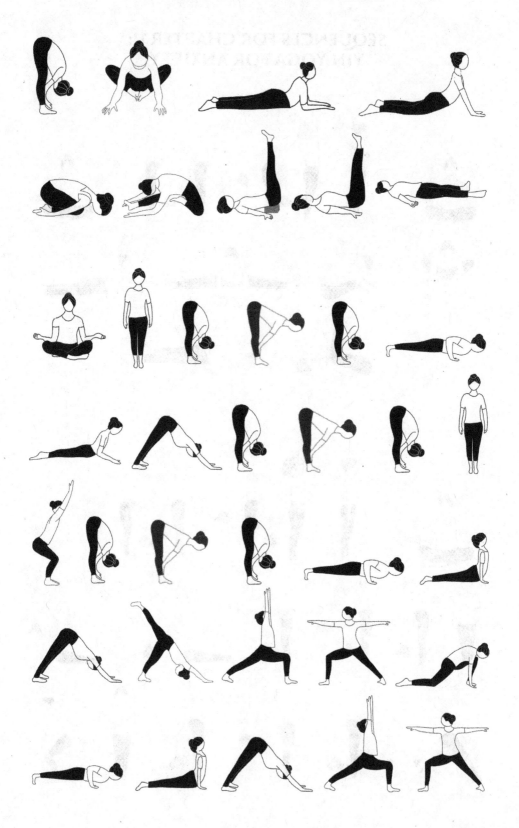

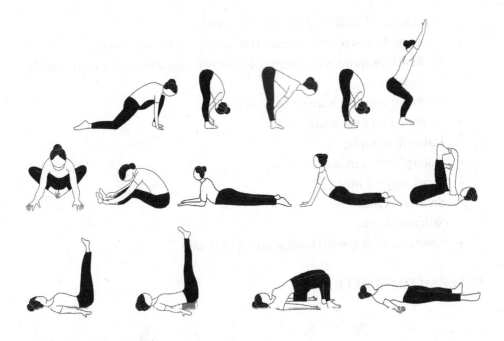

BEGINNER SEQUENCE

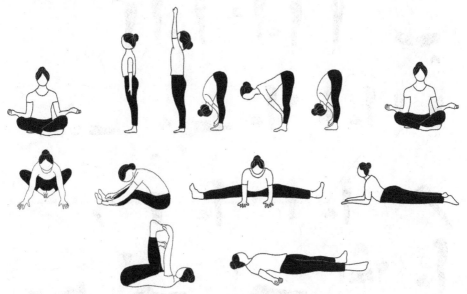

- Coherent breathing (standing or seated)—5 min. (If standing, can add Sun Salutation arms, breathing in to a count of 4 as arms raise overhead; breathing out to a count of 4 as arms release down by sides)
- 3-part breath (*dirgha pranayama*) with *ujjayi* sound (standing or seated)—2 min.
- Half Sun Salutations (3 rounds)—3 min.

- Start in Mountain Pose. Fold forward
- Bring hands to shins with a flat back. Fold forward again
- Reach arms back up keeping knees soft and come back in Mountain Pose
- Bring arms back down by your sides
- Come down to seated—1 min.
- Butterfly—2 min.
- Caterpillar—2 min.
- Dragonfly—2 min.
- Sphinx—5 min.
- Stirrup—2 min.
- *Savasana* with guided body scan—5 to 15 min.

INTERMEDIATE SEQUENCE

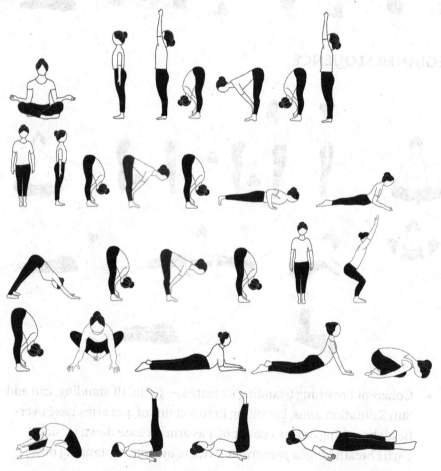

- Coherent breathing (standing or seated)—10 min.

- 3-part breath with *ujjayi* sound—2 min.
- Gentle *kapalabhati*—2 min.
- Half Sun Salutations (see description in beginner sequence) or option to move into full Sun Salutations (3 rounds)—6 min.
- Sun Salutation A series:
  - Standing Forward Fold to Jack-Knife/Flat; return to Forward Fold
  - Plank (lower to floor; option to set knees down)
  - Rise up into low Cobra; hug elbows in close to rib cage and draw chest up
  - Press back into Down Dog
  - Walk feet to hands, Forward Fold, Jack-Knife, Forward Fold
  - Reach arms up and come back into Mountain with hands in prayer position at the heart
  - Chair pose (option to add chair pose with twist to each side by hooking elbow across the body to opposite outside knee)—1 min.
- Forward Fold—30 seconds
- Butterfly—5 min.
- Sphinx or Seal—5 min.
- Child—1 min.
- Half Butterfly/Half Dragonfly—10 min. total (5 min. per side)
- Legs Up the Wall or Hip Stand with block—5 min.
- *Savasana* with *metta* (lovingkindness)—5 to 15 min.

ADVANCED SEQUENCE

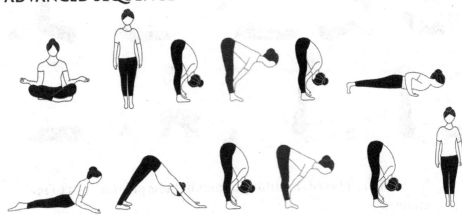

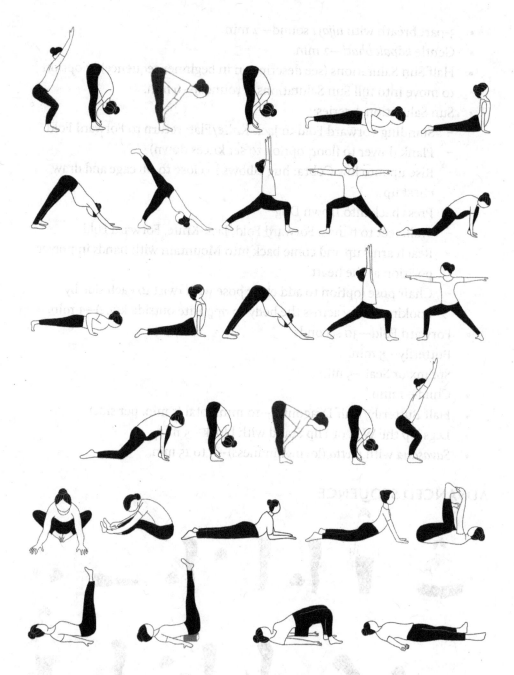

- Meditation (coherent breathing or mindfulness of breath)—5 to 15 minutes
- 3-part breath with *ujjayi* sound—2 min.
- *Kapalabhati*—option for *bhastrika* (Bellows Breath)—2 min.
- Sun Salutation A series (repeat 3 times)—6 min.

- Sun Salutation B series (repeat 3 times; with option for Warrior 1 & 2)—8 min.
  - Begin in Chair pose with hands in prayer position at the heart
  - Forward Fold to Jack-Knife/Flat Back; return to Forward Fold
  - Plank—lower to floor (option to set knees down)—Cobra
  - Press back into Down Dog
  - Extend right leg behind (Three-Legged Dog)
  - Step forward with right leg and come into Warrior 1 (arms extended overhead, right knee bent; left leg straight with heel on or off the floor)
  - Square hips to side of room for Warrior 2 with right knee still bent (arms extended level with ground, palms facing down, gaze over right arm)
  - Cartwheel the arms down and lower hands on either side of the right foot as the left foot steps back into a low lunge. Then step the right foot back to meet the left foot and come into plank pose
  - Plank—lower to floor (option to set knees down)—Cobra
  - Press back into Down Dog
  - Extend left leg behind (Three-Legged Dog)
  - Step forward with left leg and come into Warrior 1 (arms extended overhead, left knee bent, right leg straight with heel on or off the floor)
  - Square hips to the side of the room for Warrior 2 with left knee still bent (arms extended out level with the ground, palms facing down, gaze over the left arm)
  - Cartwheel the arms down and lower hands on either side of the left foot as the right foot steps back into a low lunge
  - Step right leg forward to meet left
  - Forward Fold to Jack-Knife to Forward Fold
  - Chair pose
- Butterfly—5 min.
- Caterpillar—5 min.
- Sphinx—5 min.
- Seal—5 min.
- Stirrup—5 min.
- Legs Up the Wall or Hip Stand with block or Supported Bridge with block—5 min.
- *Savasana* with yoga *nidra*—5 to 15 min.

SEQUENCES FOR CHAPTER 12: YIN YOGA FOR PTSD

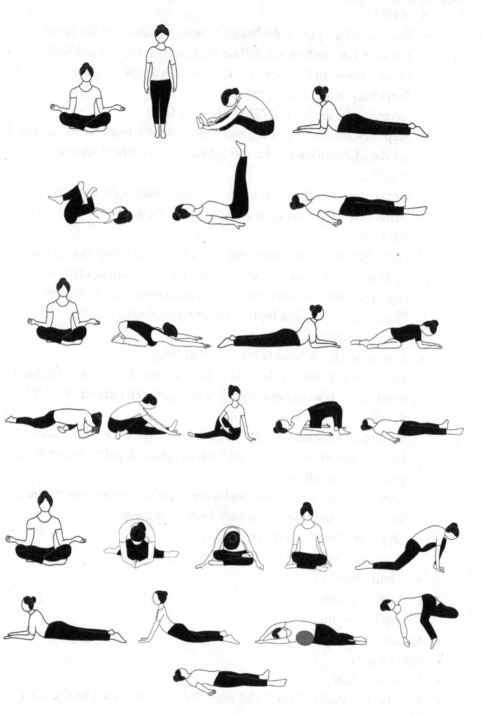

PRANAYAMA SEQUENCE

- 1:1 ratio breath (coherent breathing)—5 min.

Create a natural rhythm and flow with the breath that feels easy and deep. Match the inhale and exhale (working up to a count of 4 on the inhale and 4 on the exhale).

- Cellular breath—2 min. (with optional *ujjayi* breath: constricting the back of the throat and continuing to breathe fully in and out of the nose)

Now imagine the whole body is being breathed. Every cell is receiving oxygen from the breath, creating a sense of health and vitality.

BEGINNER SEQUENCE (YIN POSES MAY BE HELD FROM 2 TO 5 MIN., OR AS APPROPRIATE)

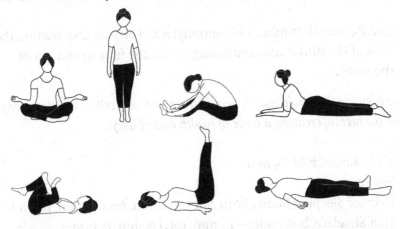

- Mindfulness of the breath, body, emotions, changing phenomena (four foundations of mindfulness)—up to 2 min. each
- 3-part breath (*dirgha pranayama* with *ujjayi* sound (standing or seated))—2 min.
- Caterpillar—2 to 5 min.
- Sphinx—2 to 5 min.
- Figure Four (on back or option to use wall)—2 to 5 min. (on each side)
- Legs Up the Wall—2 to 5 min.
- *Savasana* with option for yoga *nidra*—5 to 15 min.

INTERMEDIATE SEQUENCE (YIN POSES MAY BE HELD UP TO 5 MIN., OR AS APPROPRIATE)

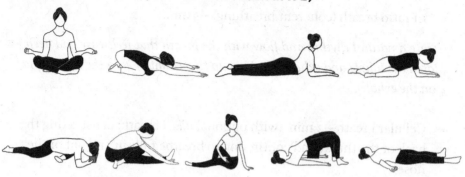

- 1:1 ratio breath (coherent breathing)—5 min.

Create a natural rhythm and flow with the breath that feels easy and deep. Match the inhale and exhale (working up to a count of 4 on the inhale and 4 on the exhale).

- Cellular breath (2 min., with optional *ujjayi* breath: constricting the back of the throat and continuing to breathe fully in and out of the nose)

Now imagine the whole body is being breathed. Every cell is receiving oxygen from the breath, creating a sense of health and vitality.

- Wide-Knee Child—5 min.
- Sphinx—5 min.
- Deer (or Sleeping Swan), both sides—10 min. total (5 min. per side)
- Half Shoelace, both sides—10 min. total (5 min. per side)
- Seated Twist, both sides—10 min. total (5 min. per side)
- Supported Bridge—5 min.
- *Savasana* with yoga *nidra*—5 to 15 min.

ADVANCED SEQUENCE (YIN POSES MAY BE HELD UP TO 5 MIN., OR AS APPROPRIATE)

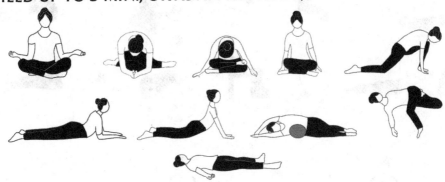

- Meditation (coherent breathing or mindfulness of breath)—5 to 15 min.
- 3-part breath with *ujjayi* sound—2 min.
- Alternate nostril breathing—2 to 5 minutes
- Shoelace, can add lateral stretch (side-bending); (modification: Figure Four)
- Square (modification: sitting cross-legged)
- Dragon, option to deepen hip opener by rolling outside edge of front foot pinky toe side with front knee remaining low to the ground and come down on elbows or rest on a bolster or block
- Sphinx or Seal
- Side-Lying Banana (using bolster/blanket)
- Cat Pull
- *Savasana* with yoga *nidra*—5 to 15 min.

SEQUENCES FOR CHAPTER 13: YIN YOGA AND TRAUMATIC BRAIN INJURY

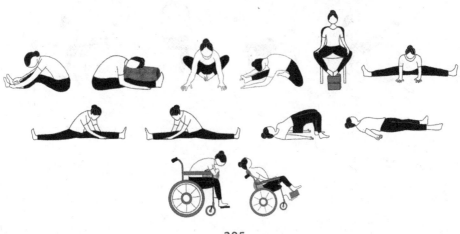

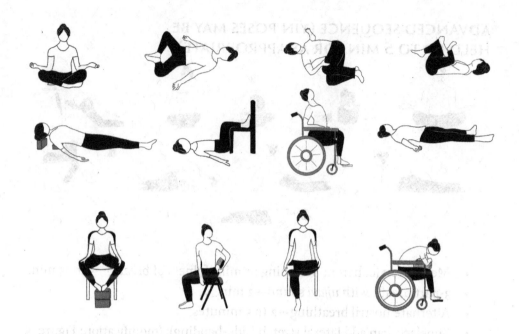

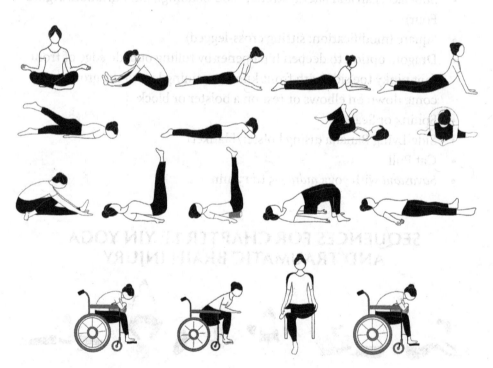

BEGINNER SEQUENCE

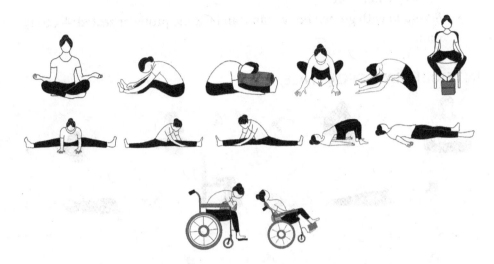

These poses can be done seated in a wheelchair or on the floor:

- Equal breathing: Begin by breathing in and counting 1 on inhale and breathing out and counting 2 on the exhale. Eyes can be open or closed. Invite a sense of curiosity and kindness into the breath
- Caterpillar (Seated Forward Fold)—1 to 2 min.
  - Modifications can include using bolster to hug or blankets under knees if seated on the floor
  - In wheelchair, gently folding over knees, place a pillow in lap
- Butterfly pose—1 to 2 min.
  - Can do one side at a time or side that has appropriate range of motion for Half Butterfly, propping with blocks or blankets as needed
  - In wheelchair, bring knees apart with feet coming toward each other; can use arms to support the knees
- Dragonfly—1 to 2 min.
  - Can do one side at a time or side that has appropriate range of movement for Half Dragonfly, propping by placing blanket under hips and under knees
  - In wheelchair, walk feet out if possible, so there is some sensation in the inner leg(s); use hands on either thigh to provide more sensation, pressing legs away
- Supported Bridge—1 to 2 min.
  - Use bolster, blankets, or other soft supports under back

- In wheelchair, place blanket or pillow behind lower back for gentle back extension
- *Savasana* with guided body scan (can be done prone or seated)—5 to 15 min.

INTERMEDIATE SEQUENCE

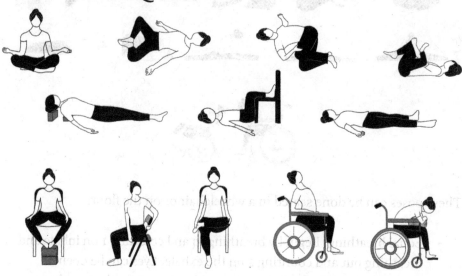

- Equal breathing—2 min. (optional: Increase to count of 4 on inhale; count of 4 on exhale)
- 3-part breath with *ujjayi* sound—2 min.
- Reclining Butterfly/Butterfly in chair—5 min.
- Reclining Twist (one or both sides if available)—10 min. total (5 min. per side)
  - In wheelchair, Seated Twist (to one or both sides if available)
- Reclining Figure Four (one or both sides if available)—10 min. total (5 min. per side)
  - In wheelchair, seated Figure Four (one or both sides if available)
- Supported Fish (bolster under back just below shoulders; block underneath head)—5 min.
  - In wheelchair, gently arch back and stay in this extension by placing a pillow or block against mid-upper back
- Legs Up on Bolster or Chair—5 min.
  - In wheelchair, gentle Forward Fold reaching arms down toward knees
- *Savasana* with *metta* (lovingkindness)

ADVANCED SEQUENCE

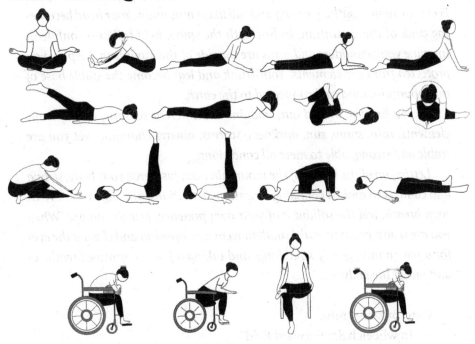

- Coherent breathing with an option to hold breath for a count of 4 after the inhale and suspend breath out and hold out for a count of 2 on the out-breath:
  - *Inhale 1, 2, 3, 4, hold 1, 2, 3, 4, exhale 1, 2, 3, 4, hold out 1, 2*
  - Repeat 10 times or as tolerated
- Single side nostril breathing: Breathe in through the left nostril, breathe out through the left nostril
  - Repeat 5 times
  - Opposite side 5 rounds
- Mountain meditation (visualization)

MOUNTAIN MEDITATION SCRIPT

Sit up and find a position where you can stay alert, upright, and stable. Support your body in any way that would make it more comfortable (sitting on a blanket or cushion, propping the knees or hips with a soft support).

Now bring to mind an image of a beautiful mountain, perhaps one that you have visited or seen in a book or movie. Appreciate its beauty and strength. Notice if your mountain has snow covering it, or whether it is covered with trees or rocks. What is the weather like? Are there are other natural wonders close by?

Now imagine that your body is the mountain, strong, calm, and stable. Feel your spine lengthen, strong and tall like a mountain. Your head becomes the peak of the mountain, in line with the spine, held tall and confident. Imagine your shoulders and arms are the side of the mountain, keeping you protected from the elements. Your trunk and legs become the stable base of the mountain, solid and connected to the earth.

As you breathe in and out, imagine the different seasons, the different elements, rain, snow, sun, darkness, storms; always changing, yet you are stable and strong, able to meet all conditions.

Letting go of the image of the mountain now, just sense your body, strong and calm, even amidst changing sensations, situations, and difficulties. With each breath, feel the solidness of your own presence, just as you are. When you are ready, begin to make small movements, opening and closing the eyes for a few rounds, gently stretching, and taking a few integrative breaths in and out of the body.

- Caterpillar—5 min.
    - In wheelchair: Forward Fold
- Baby Cobra-Sphinx-Seal—1 min. each
    - In wheelchair: Seated Cobra with arms bent at sides
- Single leg extensions in prone position—5 repetitions each side, if possible
    - In wheelchair: Single leg extensions
- Crocodile (resting prone with head on forearms for support)—2 min.
    - In wheelchair: Forward Fold
- Figure Four (reclining or seated)—10 min. total (5 min. per side)
- Shoelace (reclining or seated) crossing one knee on top of the other, drawing feet in by reaching for opposite foot using hands or yoga strap)—10 min. total (5 min. per side)
    - Can modify by doing Seated Half Shoelace or Reclining Half Shoelace
- Legs Up the Wall, or Hip Stand with block, or Supported Bridge with block—5 min.
- *Savasana* with yoga *nidra* or Light Stream meditation—5 to 15 min.

SEQUENCES FOR CHAPTER 14:
YIN YOGA FOR SCHIZOPHRENIA

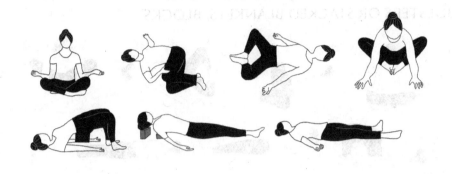

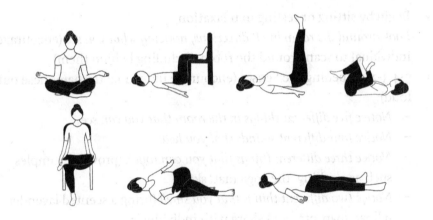

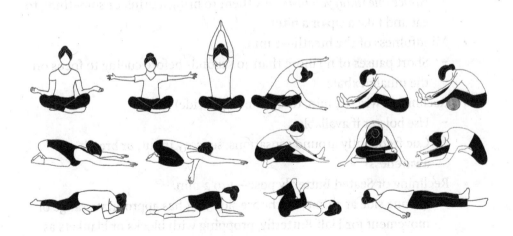

BEGINNER SEQUENCE (GROUNDING AND ORIENTING PRACTICE)
RESTING IN BED OR ON FLOOR; PROPS: BOLSTERS OR STACKED BLANKETS, BLOCKS

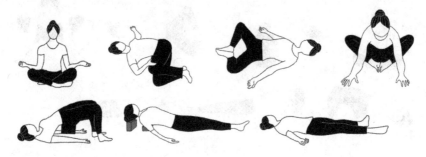

- Begin by sitting or resting in relaxation
- *Look around the room in all directions, noticing what you see* (encourage individual to scan around the room, including behind them)
- 5-4-3-2-1 Opening the Senses (encourage individual to share these out loud):
  - *Notice five different things in the room that you can see*
  - *Notice four different sounds that you hear*
  - *Notice three different things that you can touch* (provide examples, such as clothing, the yoga mat, skin)
  - *Notice two different things that you smell* (bring a scented lavender pillow, soap, etc., and share with individuals)
  - *Notice one thing you taste* (ask them to bring a drink or something to eat and take a sip or a bite)
- Mindfulness of the breath—2 min.
  - Short pauses of no more than 30 seconds before cueing to focus on the inhale/exhale
- Reclining Twist—4 min. total (2 min. per side)
  - Use bolster if available
  - Cue frequently around sensations, sensory input, or breath awareness
- Reclining or Seated Butterfly pose—1 to 2 min.
  - Do one side at a time, or choose side that has appropriate range of movement for Half Butterfly, propping with blocks or blankets as needed
  - Cue frequently around sensations, sensory input, or breath awareness

- Supported Bridge—1 to 2 min.
  - Use bolster, blankets, or other soft supports under back
  - Cue frequently around sensations, sensory input, or breath awareness
- Supported Fish—1 to 2 min.
  - Use blocks or bolster under shoulders and block or blankets under back of head
  - Cue frequently around sensations, sensory input, or breath awareness
- *Savasana* with brief guided body scan—5 min.
  - Can ask individual to move each body part rather than just "feel" to help them make more direct contact with their body

INTERMEDIATE SEQUENCE (GROUNDING AND ORIENTING PRACTICE)
RECLINING OR SEATED

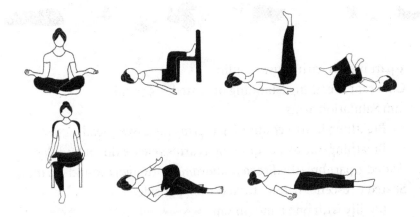

- Mindfulness of the breath—2 min. (gradual increase of space between cueing)
- Introduce 3-part breath with *ujjayi* sound—1 to 2 min.
- Legs up on Bolster, Chair, or Wall—2 to 5 min.
- Figure Four (one or both sides if possible)—4 to 10 min. total (2 to 5 min. per side)
  - Offer Seated Figure Four (one or both sides if available)
  - Transition to going through whole variation, gently pulling in opposite leg by reaching arms around lower hamstring or using yoga strap
- Twisted Root—10 min. total (5 min. per side)

- Use bolster/blanket between knees and/or on side where knees are being supported
- *Savasana* with *metta* (lovingkindness)

ADVANCED SEQUENCE (GROUNDING AND ORIENTING PRACTICE)
SEATED ON FLOOR OR IN CHAIR

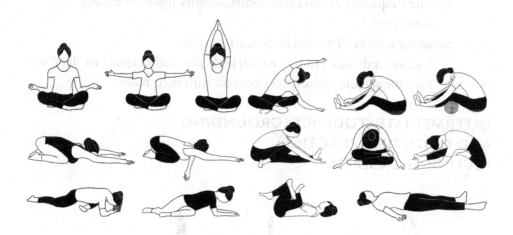

- 3-part breath with *ujjayi*—2 min.
- Coherent breathing (standing or seated)—5 min.
- Sun Salutation arms
  - Breathing in to a count of 4 as arms raise over head
  - Breathing out to a count of 4 as arms release down by sides
- Seated 3-part breath: *dirgha pranayama* with *ujjayi* sound—2 min.
- Seated Crescent—2 min. total (1 min. per side)
  - Modify with one hand on hip
- Caterpillar to Caterpillar with bolster—5 min.
- Wide-Knee Child—5 min.
  - Option to add twist to each side
- Half Shoelace—10 min. total (5 min. per side)
  - Option for support under hip and opposite knee
- Open Square (variation: Half Butterfly)—10 min. total (5 min. per side)
- Sleeping Swan or Deer—10 min. total (5 min. per side)
- Figure Four
- *Savasana* with option for body scan with progressive muscle relaxation

PROGRESSIVE MUSCLE RELAXATION SCRIPT

As you come to the end of practice, become aware of your breathing once more. Notice how your abdomen rises and falls with each breath. Let your breathing rhythm return to normal...and relax...

During this relaxation, I will ask you to tense various muscles throughout your body. Please do this without straining. You do not need to exert yourself, just contract each muscle firmly but gently as you breathe in. If you feel uncomfortable at any time, you can simply relax and breathe normally.

Bring your awareness to your feet and toes. Breathe in deeply through your nose, and as you do, gradually curl your toes down and tense the muscles in the soles of your feet. Hold your breath for just a few seconds and then release the muscles in your feet as you breathe out. Feel the tension in your feet wash away as you exhale. Notice how different your feet feel when they are tensed and when they are relaxed. Take another deep breath in, tense the muscles in the soles of your feet, and hold this position for a few seconds. Now release. Feel yourself relaxing more and more deeply with each breath. Your whole body is becoming heavier, softer and more relaxed as each moment passes.

Now bring your awareness to your lower legs, to your calf muscles. As you draw in a nice, deep breath, point your toes up toward your knees and tighten these muscles. Hold for just a moment, and then let those muscles go limp as you exhale. Once again, draw in a deep breath...and tighten your calf muscles. Hold for a few seconds, and then let it all go. Feel your muscles relax, and feel the tension washing away with your out-breath.

In a moment, you will tense the muscles in the front of your thighs. If you are lying down, you can do this by trying to straighten your legs. You'll feel the muscles pulling your kneecap upwards. If you are seated, you can tense these muscles by pushing your heels down onto the floor. Take a deep breath in, and tense the muscles in your thighs. Hold for just a moment, and then release everything. As you do this, the blood flow to your muscles increases, and you may notice a warm, tingling sensation. Enjoy this feeling of soothing relaxation in your thighs. Again, breathe in deeply and tighten your thigh muscles. Hold for a moment. Now release. Focus on letting your muscles go.

Draw in a nice, deep breath and gradually tighten the muscles in your buttocks. Hold this contraction for a few seconds, and then release your breath. Feel the tension leaving your muscles. Feel them relaxing completely. Once more, breathe in deeply and tighten the muscles in your buttocks. Hold for a moment. Now release them. You are becoming more and more deeply relaxed. Take another breath, and this time, gradually tighten all the muscles in your legs, from your feet to your buttocks. Do this in whatever way feels natural and comfortable to you. Hold it...and now release all these large, strong muscles. Enjoy the sensation of release as you become even more deeply relaxed.

Now bring your awareness to your stomach. Draw in a deep breath and then tighten these muscles. Now release your breath and let your muscles relax. Notice the sensation of relief that comes from letting go. Once again, draw in a deep breath and then tighten your stomach muscles. Hold for a few seconds...and then let them relax as you exhale and release all tension.

Bring your awareness to the muscles in your back. As you slowly breathe in, arch your back slightly and tighten these muscles, being careful not to strain or create too much sensation. Now release your breath and let your muscles relax. Again, draw in a deep breath and then tighten your back muscles. Hold for a few seconds...and then let them relax and release.

Now give your attention to your shoulder muscles and the muscles in your neck. As you slowly draw in a deep breath, pull your shoulders up toward your ears and squeeze these muscles firmly. Now breathe out completely and allow your contracted muscles to relax. Again, pull your shoulders up toward your ears and squeeze these muscles firmly. Now feel the tension subside as you relax and breathe out. Feel the heaviness in your body now. Enjoy the feeling. Feel yourself becoming heavier and heavier. Feel yourself becoming more and more deeply relaxed. You are calm and at ease.

Now it's time to let go of tension in your arms and hands. Let's start with your upper arms. As you breathe in, raise your wrists toward your shoulders and tighten the muscles in your upper arms. Hold that breath and that contraction for just a moment...and then gently lower your arms and breathe all the way out. You may feel a warm, burning sensation in your muscles when you tighten them. Feel how relaxing it is to release that tightness and to breathe away all tension. As you curl your upper arms again, tighten the muscles as you breathe in. Breathe in deeply. Now relax your arms and breathe out. Now bring your awareness to your forearms. As you breathe in, curl your hands inward as though you are trying to touch the inside of your elbows with your fingertips. Now feel the tension subside as you relax and breathe out. Again, take a deep breath in, and tighten the muscles in your forearms. Hold it for a moment, and then release them. Feel the tension washing away. Now, take another breath in and tightly clench your fists. When you have finished breathing in, hold for just a few seconds, and then release. Notice any feelings of buzzing or throbbing. Your hands are becoming very soft and relaxed. Take another deep breath in and clench your fists again. Hold for just a few seconds, and then release. Let your fingers completely relax. Your arms and hands are feeling heavy and relaxed. Take a couple of nice long slow breaths now, and just relax. Feel yourself slipping even deeper into a state of complete rest.

Now tighten the muscles in your face by squeezing your eyes shut and clenching your lips together. As you do, breathe in fully. Hold it...now breathe out and relax all your facial muscles. Feel your face softening. Once more, breathe in deeply while you scrunch the muscles in your eyes and lips...and release. Now bring your awareness to the muscles in your jaw. Take a deep breath in, and then open your mouth as wide as you can. Feel your jaw muscles stretching and tightening. Now, exhale and allow your mouth to gently close. Again, fill your lungs with air and then open your mouth wide. Now let your mouth relax, and let your breath release all the way out. You are now completely relaxed from the tips of your toes to the top of your head. Feel your whole body relaxed and at ease. When you are ready, begin to gently open and close your eyes a few times, letting your eyes adjust to being awake. Make some small gentle movements with your fingers and toes and then begin to move slowly into a comfortable seated position.

ENDNOTES

1   Brown, A. (2014) 'How many breaths do you take each day?' https://blog.epa.gov/2014/04/28/how-many-breaths-do-you-take-each-day.

2   Brown, R.P., and Gerbarg, P.L. (2012) *The Healing Power of the Breath.* Boston, MA: Shambhala Press.

3   Brown, R.P., and Gerbarg, P.L. (2020) *Breath-Body-Mind™ Level-1 Teacher Training Manual.* New York: Breath-Body-Mind LLC.

4   Linehan, M. (2015) *DBT Skills Training Handouts and Worksheets* (2nd ed.). New York: Guilford Press.

5   Van Dijk, S. (2012) *DBT Made Simple.* Oakland, CA: New Harbinger.

CONCLUSION

In my clinical work, nearly every client describes feelings of anxiety and over-whelm. Physical and mental fatigue are a daily experience. Hearing their stories, I am struck by how few tools people actually have to work with these uncomfortable symptoms.

Fortunately, as I described in the many heroic stories of my clients throughout this book, yin yoga can be an important part of a tool kit for mental health and physical wellness. I also included many studies throughout this book on the growing body of research around yoga for mental health. These studies demonstrate the benefit of integrating yoga to support healing and recovery from a variety of psychiatric and neurocognitive conditions.

By incorporating yin yoga, mindfulness meditation, and principles of positive psychology, individuals can quickly and effectively learn how to regulate their nervous system response to stress and begin a journey of self-care. For yoga therapists and mental health clinicians, teaching clients how to use the simple physical practices of yin yoga can become an important part of the therapeutic process. These practices can strengthen the therapeutic alliance between the clinician and client using inquiry, mindfulness and compassion and provide an *in vivo* opportunity for the client to experience ease, joy, and acceptance.

INDEX

Vadiraja, H.S. *et al.* 119
vagus nerve 46–8
Vahratian, A. *et al.* 11
Vancampfort, D. *et al.* 173
Van der Kolk, B.A. 141, 143, 145
Van Reekum, R. *et al.* 155
Varambally, S. *et al.* 173–4
Vedamurthachar, A. *et al.* 119
vibrational breathing (*bhramari*) 74
vipassana (self-observation) 71–2
virtue ethics 58
Visceglia, E. 28, 173

Wallace, Alan 92, 94–6
Wallace, R.K. *et al.* 75
Watson, John 129
The Web That Has No Weaver (Kaptchuk) 61
Weforum 126
Wehring, H.J. 169
West, J. *et al.* 144
"What" Skills script 107–8, 267
A Whole-Life Path (Kramer) 82
Wide-Knee Child (Frog) pose 63, 212–13, 246–8
"window of tolerance" (Siegel) 47–8, 50, 113
Wise Mind script 107–8, 266–7
Wood Becomes Water: Chinese Medicine in Everyday Life (Reichstein) 61
Woodman, M. 40
World Health Organization 114, 155, 168
Wykes, T. *et al.* 172
Wynn, G.H. 143

yamas 58
The Yamas and Niyamas (Adele) 58
yang organs 62, 63–4
"yin" 30–2
yin organs 62, 63–4
yin sensation scale 19–20
Yinsights (Clark) 21
yin yoga
    benefits (overview) and challenges 30–2
    concept described 15–16
    see other yoga forms 16–18
    ethical practices of 58

functional alignment approach 34–5
general principles 18–23
history of 18
and intention 60–1
and interoception awareness 36–9
key characteristics 16–18
key treatment combinations 131–2
mechanisms of action (psychiatric conditions) 144, 173–4
pace of 40
safe place/inner resource 54–5, 59–60, 255–6
and self-inquiry 39–40
social connections of 58–9
use of props 17, 35–6
with ANTs 105–6
with breath awareness and enhancement 69–76
with cognitive behavioral approaches 98–110
with DBT 106–8
with Eightfold Path practices 79–85
with Internal Family Systems (IFS) therapy 110
with lovingkindness (Four Heart) practices 65–6, 87–97, 178, 260–1, 279, 288, 294
with *Qi* flow and the meridians 61–4
The Yin Yoga Kit (Mithoefer) 185
Yin Yoga Principles and Practices (Grilley) 185
yoga instruction giving 16–17
Yoga as Medicine: The Yogic Prescription for Health and Healing (McCall) 28–9
yoga *nidra* 31–2, 54, 120
    for PTSD 145–6
yoga poses 185–245
    key principles 19–23
    length of hold time 16, 19
    skeletal limitations and functional alignment 34–5
    use of props 17, 35–6
    using different versions of 34–5
    Banana-Asana (Reclining Side Bend) 113, 186–7

Bound Angle/Butterfly 24, 63, 136, 145, 152, 190–2
Breath Of Joy 132, 187–8, 254
Cat/Cow 194–6
Caterpillar (Seated Forward Fold) 196–7
Cat Pull 192–3
Child 33, 198–9
Crescent Moon 240–1
Dangle/Standing Forward Fold 199–200
Deer 201–2
Down Dog 202–4
Dragon 64, 206–7
Dragonfly 63–4, 204–6
Extended Tabletop 242
Figure Four 208–9
Fish 209–10
Five-Pointed Star 211–12
Frog/Wide-Knee Child 63, 212–13, 246–8
Goddess 214–15
Half-Moon 240–1
Happy Baby (Stirrup) pose 35, 138, 215–16
Knees Into Chest 217–18
Legs Up the Wall 42, 49–50, 218–19
Meditation 220–2, 249–52
Mountain 222–3
Pigeon 233–4
Puppy (Quarter Dog) 63, 64, 223–4
Saddle 225–6
Savasana 53, 60, 85, 226–7, 259, 261–3, 278–9
Sphinx 63, 124, 236–7
Square 237–8
Squat 238–9
Supported Bridge 87, 152, 188–90
Tabletop 241–2
Thread The Needle 243–4
Twisted Root 244–5
see also yin yoga
Yoga and the Quest for the True Self (Cope) 73
Yoga Sutras of Patanjali 25, 58, 73

Zeng, X. *et al.* 178
Zuo, X.L. *et al.* 57